OTHER VOLUMES IN
EXERCISES IN DIAGNOSTIC RADIOLOGY

Published

ADVANCED EXERCISES IN DIAGNOSTIC RADIOLOGY

Published

Forthcoming

EXERCISES IN DIAGNOSTIC RADIOLOGY

8

DIAGNOSTIC ULTRASOUND

BARBARA BOWLING GOSINK, M.D.

Chief, Ultrasound Section, Veterans
Administration Hospital; Assistant
Professor of Radiology in Residence
University of California, San Diego

LUCY FRANK SQUIRE, M.D.

Professor of Radiology, Downstate Medical
Center, Brooklyn, New York; Consultant
in Radiology, Massachusetts General
Hospital, Boston

W. B. SAUNDERS COMPANY · PHILADELPHIA · LONDON · TORONTO

W. B. Saunders Company: West Washington Square
Philadelphia, Pa.   19105

1 St. Anne's Road
Eastbourne, East Sussex BN21 3UN, England

833 Oxford Street
Toronto, Ontario M8Z 5T9, Canada

Library of Congress Cataloging in Publication Data (Revised)

Main entry under title:

Exercises in diagnostic radiology.

CONTENTS: 1.   The chest.—2.   The abdomen.—3.   Bone.
[etc.]

1. Diagnosis, Radioscopic.   I. Squire, Lucy Frank. [DNLM:
   1. Emergencies—Programmed texts. WN100 S774fa v. 7]

RC78.E89   616.07'57   74–113034

Exercises in Diagnostic Radiology—
Volume 8 Diagnostic Ultrasound   ISBN   0-7216-4176-8

Print No.:   9   8   7   6   5   4   3   2

PREFACE

This volume is an introduction to the relatively new science (and art) of diagnostic ultrasound. The purpose of this text is to guide the reader through various clinical problems which are amenable to solution or clarification by the use of ultrasound. In the chapters devoted to abdominal and pelvic B-scanning, the complementary relationships of ultrasound to other imaging techniques, such as nuclear medicine and conventional radiography, will be established.

Although the basic principles underlying generation of the ultrasonic beam were discovered late in the 19th century (13 years before the discovery of x-ray), for many years ultrasound was considered a curiosity, useful only in dog whistles. Bats and dolphins, of course, were more imaginative. Wartime development of sonar techniques gave impetus to the study of ultrasonics. It is only in the past 10 years, however, that there has been widespread interest in medical applications of the technique.

This increasing interest in (and availability of) diagnostic ultrasound led to our realization of a need for this type of book. Although primarily geared as an introductory text for medical students, showing how diagnostic ultrasound can help to solve some common clinical problems, this book will also be helpful to others (both physicians and technologists) interested in this new discipline.

For readers who desire a more detailed consideration of the underlying principles, techniques, and applications of ultrasound we particularly recommend the following texts:

1. Eycleshymer, A. C., and Schoemaker, D. M.: *A Cross-Section Anatomy.* New York, Appleton-Century-Crofts, 1970.
2. Wells, P. N. T.: *Physical Principles of Ultrasonic Diagnosis.* New York, Academic Press, 1969.
3. Leopold, G. R., and Asher, M.: *Fundamentals of Abdominal and Pelvic Ultrasonography.* Philadelphia, W. B. Saunders Co., 1975.
4. King, D. L. (Ed.): *Diagnostic Ultrasound.* St. Louis, The C. V. Mosby Co., 1974.
5. Feigenbaum, H.: *Echocardiography.* Philadelphia, Lea & Febiger, 1972.
6. Joyner, C. R.: *Ultrasound in the Diagnosis of Cardiovascular-Pulmonary Disease.* Chicago, Year Book Medical Publishers, Inc., 1974.
7. Kobayashi, M.: *Illustrated Manual of Ultrasonography in Obstetrics and Gynecology.* Tokyo, Igaku Shoin Ltd., and Philadelphia, J. B. Lippincott Co., 1974.

Techniques of diagnostic ultrasound and applications of the modality are constantly changing. This book is a survey of the more common situations likely to be encountered in clinical practice. As in previous volumes of the Exercises, we eagerly seek suggestions and comments from our readers.

BARBARA BOWLING GOSINK, M.D.

LUCY FRANK SQUIRE, M.D.

ACKNOWLEDGMENTS

The authors wish to express their gratitude to the many people who contributed to this book. Particular mention must be made of the dedicated ultrasound technical specialists who produced studies not only of diagnostic quality, but also with esthetic appeal. Two such individuals are John R. Forsythe, senior sonographer, and Nanette E. Grandjean, both of the Veterans Administration Hospital at San Diego. Laura L. Schorzman and Margot L. Henkelmann from the University Hospital, San Diego, were also helpful in this regard.

Special thanks go to Dr. George R. Leopold of the University Hospital, whose encouragement, good humor, and advice were invaluable. Nearly all of the cases in Chapter 5 and several cases elsewhere throughout the book are from Dr. Leopold's department. Drs. Joshua Becker and Morton Schneider from the State University of New York, Downstate reviewed the entire manuscript and gave us many useful suggestions. Dr. Allen D. Johnson, Acting Chief of Cardiology, Veterans Administration Hospital at San Diego, evaluated Chapter 6 and provided some excellent critical ideas. Dr. Robert Penner reviewed the section on ophthalmology and contributed all of the photographs in that section. Dr. Leonard Gosink read the section on echoencephalography and served as a "test subject" for most of one year. We are grateful for the encouragement and enthusiasm of Dr. Folke J. Brahme.

Janet Julien and Paula Nicholas of the Medical Illustration Department, Veterans Administration Hospital at San Diego, prepared the drawings and diagrams. From the same department, Susan Brown and Robert C. Turner provided exacting photographic work. Their efforts are much appreciated.

Dorie Kehew typed and retyped multiple versions of the manuscript. W. Jane Pappas also lent herself to this task.

Mr. and Mrs. George A. Bowling are responsible for most of the more outrageous puns.

Finally, our warmest thanks go to the score of medical students who took the time to read the manuscript and offer so much useful feedback. This book is for them.

BARBARA BOWLING GOSINK
LUCY FRANK SQUIRE

CONTENTS

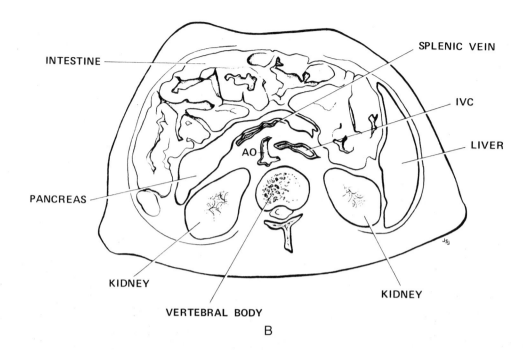

B

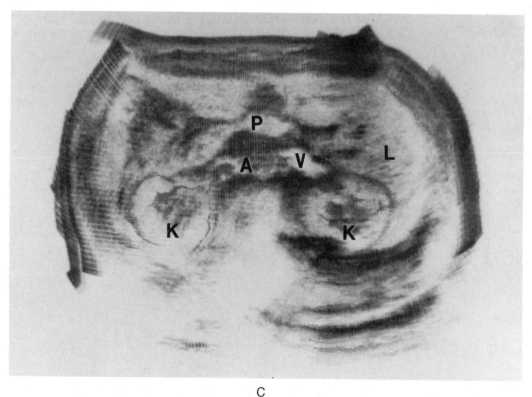

C

I. A. Color Plate: Cross section of normal cadaver obtained 8 cm. cephalad to the umbilicus. (From Leopold, G. R., and Asher, W. M.: Fundamentals of Abdominal and Pelvic Ultrasonography. Philadelphia, W. B. Saunders Co., 1974.)

B. Line drawing of cadaver.

C. Transverse ultrasound study of the abdomen at a similar level in another patient. The liver (L) in this patient is larger than in the cadaver section and extends far to the left anterior to the pancreas (P). The aorta (A) is not clearly outlined in this patient. Vena cava (V). Kidneys (K). (Retouched)

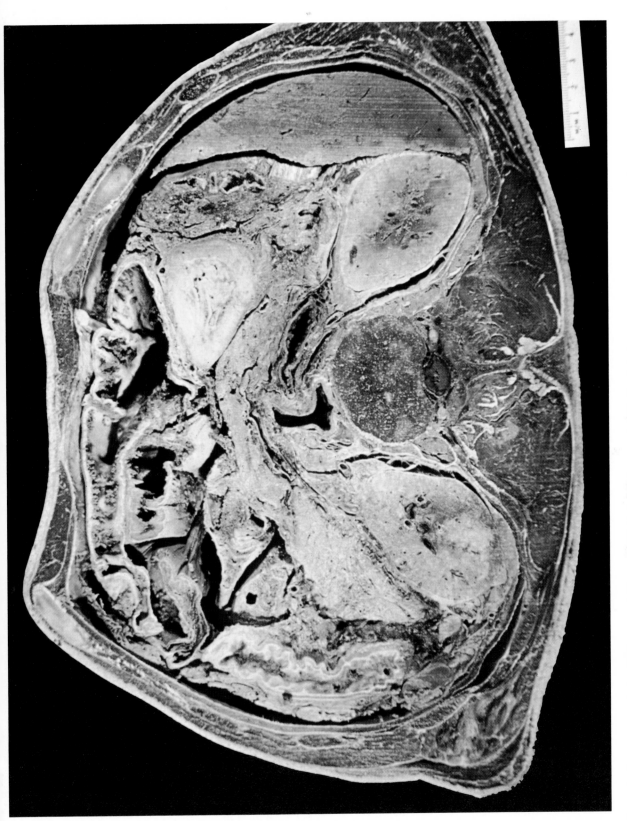

A

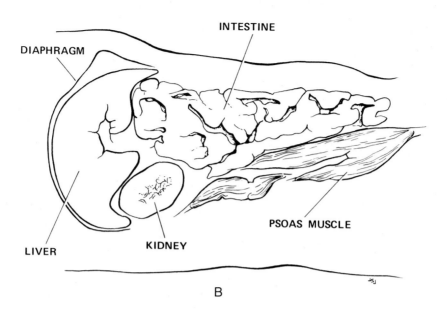

B

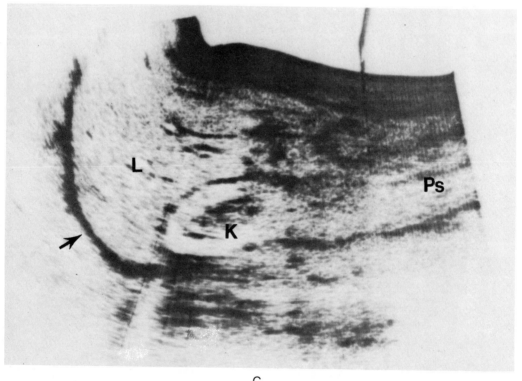

C

II. A. Color Plate: Longitudinal section of normal cadaver obtained approximately 7 cm. to the right of midline. (From Leopold, G. R., and Asher, W. M.: Fundamentals of Abdominal and Pelvic Ultrasonography. Philadelphia, W. B. Saunders Co., 1974.)

B. Line drawing of cadaver.

C. Longitudinal ultrasound scan obtained approximately 7 cm. to the right of midline. Liver (L). Kidney (K). Psoas (Ps.). Diaphragm (arrow). The umbilicus is indicated by an electronic marker.

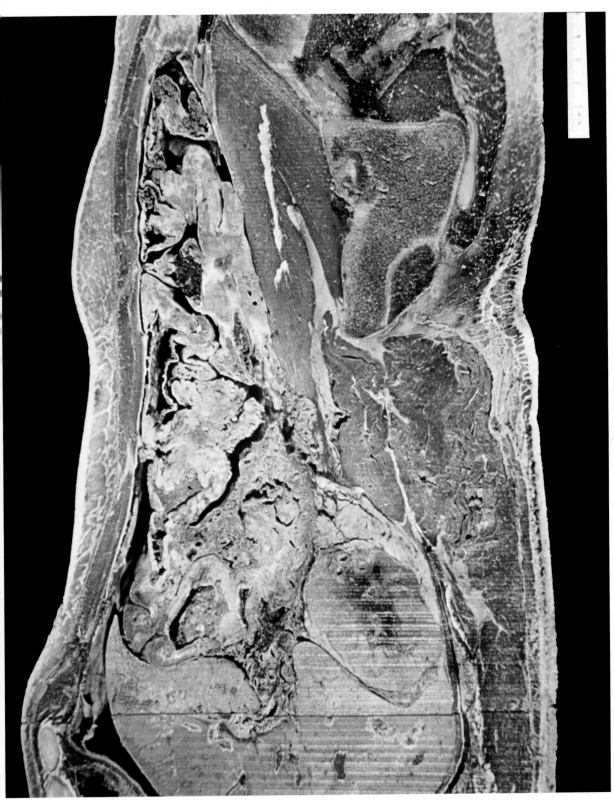

A

CHAPTER 1

GENERAL PRINCIPLES

The use of ultrasound as a tool in medical diagnosis is gaining increased acceptance in most medical centers. The chief advantages of ultrasound as a diagnostic modality are three:

1. It is a noninvasive study, causing little or no discomfort to the patient and usually requiring no special preparation.
2. It does not require the use of ionizing radiation such as x-rays. Studies to date have shown no proven adverse effects from the ultrasonic beam at the conventional power levels used for diagnosis.
3. Ultrasound is capable of providing some diagnostic information which may not be available using other noninvasive techniques.

The ultrasound beam is in many ways similar to a beam of light. It obeys the laws of optics and can (unlike x-rays) be focused, reflected, or refracted. The beam consists of high frequency sound waves generated by vibration of a piezoelectric crystal within an ultrasound transducer. The crystal vibrates in response to an electrical signal, the frequency of vibration being a function of the shape and thickness of the crystal itself. This is exactly the same principle that governs the sound of a bell. Bells of differing shapes and sizes have differing frequencies of vibration, and therefore *sound* different. For most medical applications, the frequency used is approximately 2.5 million cycles per second (2.5 megaHertz). The same crystal that transmits the ultrasonic beam also functions as a listening device. For example, a pulse of ultrasound is beamed for a fraction of a second and the crystal then "listens" during a much longer interval for the echo response. Returning sound waves (echoes) strike the transducer, producing vibrations which are transmitted as electrical signals to an oscilloscope or for storage on the screen of a cathode ray tube.

What produces these echoes? The tissues of the body vary from each other in sound-transmission characteristics (acoustic impedance). When two tissues of *differing* acoustic impedance are apposed, the ultrasonic beam will be partially reflected at the *interface* between them, returning an echo signal to the transducer. The degree of difference in acoustic impedance will determine the strength of the returning echo. Thus, if *soft tissue* lies next to *bone*, which has a very high acoustic impedance, or next to *air*, which has a very low acoustic impedance, strong interfaces will be formed, and strong echoes will be returned. On the other hand, *soft tissues* (vessel walls, septa, fat, parenchyma, etc.) *differ only slightly from one another in acoustic impedance* and the echoes that are returned from their various interfaces are relatively weak. These echoes are recorded as spikes on an oscilloscope or stored as dots on the screen of the cathode ray tube. This latter type of storage display is called a B-scan, B because the *brightness* (and size) of the dots on the screen varies with the strength of the acoustic interface.

B-Scanning

B-scan displays are used when performing studies of the abdomen, retroperitoneum, and pelvis. The orientation of the dots on the storage screen varies with the orientation of the transducer relative to the patient's body. As the transducer (attached to a rigid hinged arm, which holds it in any plane selected) is moved across a section of the patient's body, it sends a narrow, well-directed ultrasonic beam through the tissues (Figs. 1–1A and 1–1B). As this beam traverses the abdomen, it is partially reflected at various interfaces, owing to relative differences in acoustic impedance. These reflected echoes are recorded as dots, which build up an image of the section on a storage screen (Fig. 1–2). When a

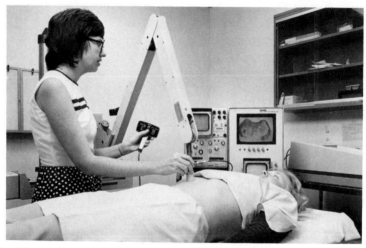

Fig. 1–1A. **Ultrasound study in progress. The operator has moved the transducer transversely across the patient's upper abdomen. This produces a picture on the storage screen. When an appropriate picture has been produced, it may be photographed or recorded on heat-sensitive paper.**

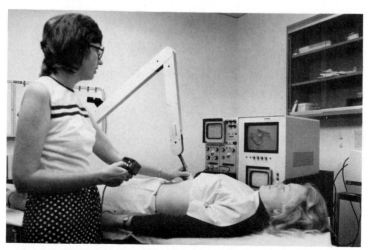

Fig. 1–1B. **Longitudinal study in progress. Now you can see the rigid hinged arm to which the transducer is attached.**

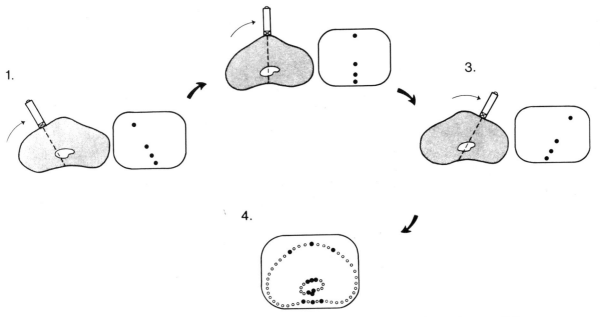

Fig. 1–2. Diagram. As the transducer is moved across the body, an image of the body section traversed is built up on the storage screen.

suitable picture has been made, it may be photographed on either Polaroid or x-ray film, or recorded on heat-sensitive paper.

It is important to remember that relatively inhomogeneous tissues, such as solid organs or masses, will generally have many weak echoes recorded within them, representing small vessels, ducts, and septae traversing the tissue. Relatively homogeneous tissues, such as fluid-filled organs or cystic lesions, show few internal echoes, even when the sensitivity of the machine is turned up very high ("high gain").

A complete study requires many pictures and may include transverse, oblique, and longitudinal sections. Just as it is difficult to visualize a loaf of bread from a single slice, an ultrasonic study also requires many "slices" for satisfactory visualization. (You *could* slice a loaf of bread longitudinally, couldn't you?) Ultrasound is similar in this respect to x-ray tomography. You would not be willing to say that a chest film was normal if all you had was a normal tomographic cut at 10 cm. from the posterior chest wall.

Space limitations require that we present only one or two pictures from each patient in this book, but you *must* remember that any finding pointed out here was necessarily verified on multiple sections in an individual patient.

Enough of these basics for now (more later). Let's see if you can *apply* these principles to some everyday objects.

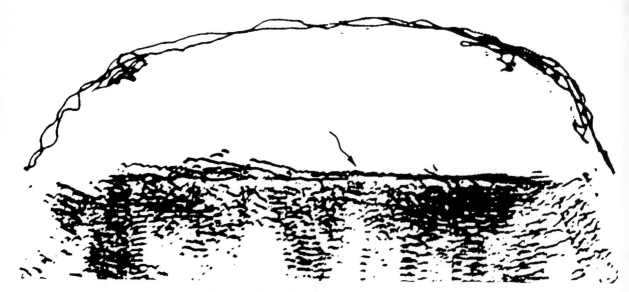

Fig. 1–3A. Echogram. Common edible.

PROBLEM

Here's an ultrasonic cross section (echogram, Fig. 1–3A) of a common edible that is particularly popular in hospital cafeterias. Is it homogeneous or inhomogeneous? Can you guess what it is?

HINT: Ignore, for the present, the many dark echoes seen at the bottom of the picture. The true posterior border of this substance is shown by the arrow.

ANSWER

Jello, of course (Fig. 1–3B)! The slightly irregular outline on the echogram is due to the difficulties inherent in working with an uncooperative (and melting) subject. Also notice the many echoes seen *beyond* the Jello, indicating that little of the sound energy was used up in traversing this homogeneous substance. Much of the energy passed through the Jello and caused strong echoes from the table beneath ("high through transmission"). Incidentally, would the plain Jello look the same on the echogram if it were in the liquid state?

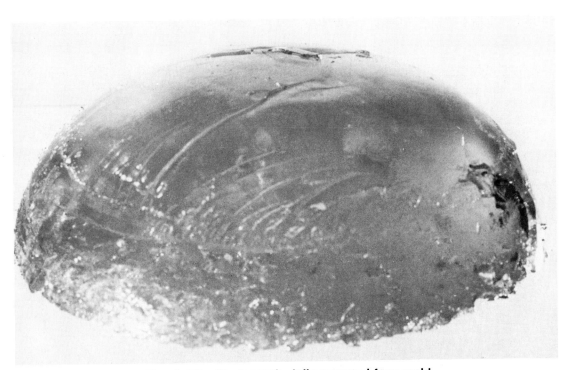

Fig. 1–3B. **Photograph. Jello removed from mold.**

Now, what do you think the echogram would look like if the Jello had fruit in it? Would there be echoes inside? *Draw* your concept of the resulting echogram on a slip of paper.

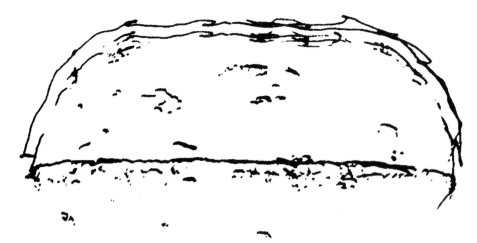

Fig. 1–4A. Echogram. Jello with fruit.

Note that many small echoes are seen within the fruit-filled Jello (Fig. 1–4A), indicating interfaces of differing acoustic impedance between fruit and Jello. Also, since more sound energy has been used up striking interfaces *within* the Jello, there is less through transmission and therefore fewer echoes beyond. (Compare with Fig. 1–3A). In the plain Jello, little beam energy was used up traversing the substance; therefore, many echoes *could* be recorded from the table beyond.

TEACHING POINT: Echograms provide information about the size, shape and *homogeneity* of structures. They do *not*, per se, tell whether a structure is cystic or solid. For instance, a fluid-filled mass containing septae or necrotic debris will have some internal echoes.

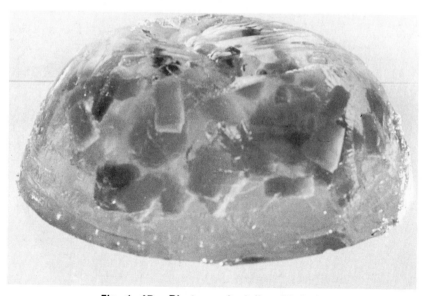

Fig. 1–4B. Photograph. Jello with fruit.

This brings us to an important difference between diagnostic ultrasound and x-ray. If we were to *x-ray* the plain and the fruit-filled Jello, do you think the pictures would look different? Of course not. X-ray cannot distinguish between various tissues of water density (such as fruit and Jello, or cysts and tumors). With diagnostic ultrasound, this distinction can easily be made.

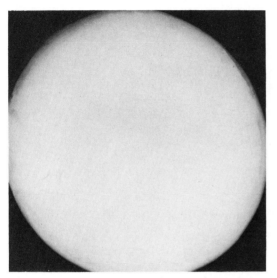

Fig. 1–5A. **X-ray. Plain Jello.**

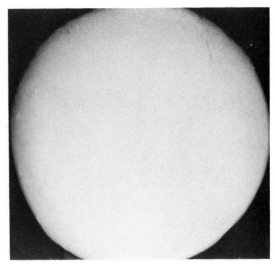

Fig. 1–5B. **X-ray. Jello with fruit.**

ANSWER TO QUESTION ON PAGE 5

Plain Jello in the liquid state would echographically look the same as plain Jello in the solid state (although the shape might differ!).

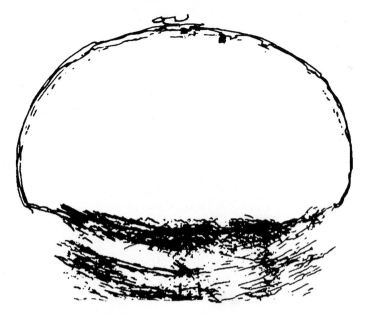

Fig. 1–6A. **Echogram. Water-filled balloon. Note the many echoes in back, indicating high through transmission.**

Figure 1–6*A* shows an echogram of a water-filled balloon (slightly flattened by lying on the table). The ultrasonic beam traversed the water easily, and the posterior surface of the balloon (most distal from the transducer) is well outlined. Also note the high through transmission beyond. These three findings (no internal echoes, sharp distal border and high through transmission) are characteristic of very homogeneous (usually fluid-filled) structures.

PROBLEM

What would an ultrasonic cross section of an air-filled balloon look like? Would you be able to outline the posterior wall?

> HINT: Air has an extremely low acoustic impedance, differing markedly from the impedances of soft tissues. Remember that it is the amount of *difference* in acoustic impedance between two adjacent structures which determines what proportion of the beam is reflected directly back to the transducer and what proportion traverses the tissue.

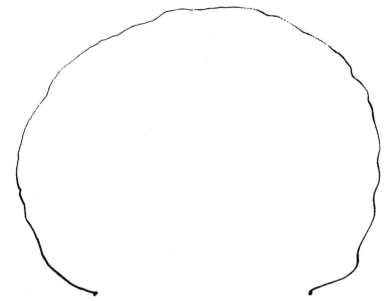

Fig. 1–6B. Echogram. Air-filled balloon. The back wall is not delineated.

ANSWERS

The acoustic impedance of air differs so markedly from that of water that almost all the sound energy is reflected back by this strong acoustic interface. Therefore, no energy can penetrate to reveal the back of the balloon (Fig. 1–6B).

Figure 1–6C shows an echogram of a water-filled balloon with an air bubble floating at the top. The air bubble interferes with visualization of a small portion of the posterior surface of the water-filled balloon.

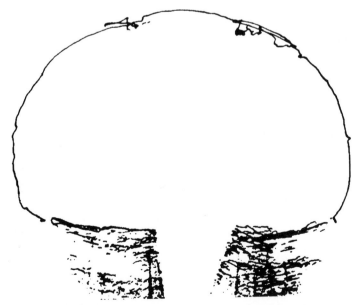

Fig. 1–6C. Echogram. Water-filled balloon with air bubble floating at top. The back surface beneath the air bubble is not delineated.

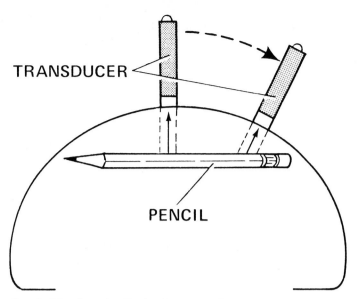

TRANSDUCER

PENCIL

Fig. 1–7A. **Longitudinal diagram. Pencil suspended in water-filled balloon. The strong acoustic interface at the water-pencil border prevents transmission of the ultrasonic beam.**

Bone and barium have a very *high* acoustic impedance in comparison to soft tissues. So does a pencil. If we were to suspend a pencil near the top of our water-filled balloon (Fig. 1–7A), what do you think the echogram would look like? Try drawing longitudinal and transverse sections yourself.

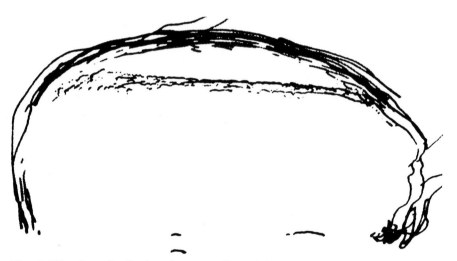

Fig. 1–7B. **Longitudinal echogram. Pencil suspended in water-filled balloon. The back surface of the balloon is not delineated because the beam could not penetrate beyond the pencil.**

Same principle: The acoustic impedance of the pencil is so different from that of the water that a strong acoustic interface is created. This interferes markedly with beam transmission, so that on the midline longitudinal section no sound energy is transmitted to the back wall of the balloon (Fig. 1–7B).

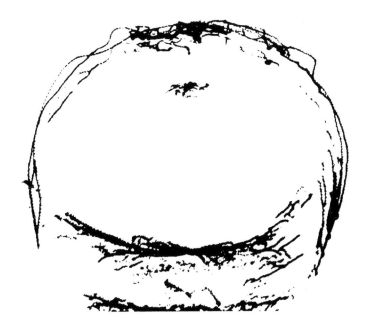

Fig. 1–8A. Transverse echogram. Pencil suspended in water-filled balloon.

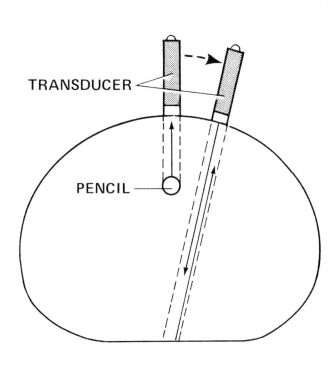

TRANSDUCER

PENCIL

Fig. 1–8B. Transverse diagram. Pencil suspended in water-filled balloon. Note how the beam is angled in from the side to delineate the back wall of the balloon beyond the pencil.

How can we see the complete posterior wall on the transverse view (Fig. 1–8A)? Easy: we cheat, angling the beam in from the side (Fig. 1–8B). This technique of angling the beam is commonly used during an echographic study to circumvent barriers such as ribs and air-filled loops of bowel.

A recent advance in ultrasonic technology has been the development of "gray scale" equipment. These units are capable of recording echoes from the parenchyma of many organs in far greater detail than was previously possible. The older (or "bistable"—i.e., recording only black and white) ultrasound machines record echoes only from interfaces that are stronger than a certain threshold (Fig. 1–9). One may *lower* this threshold by turning up the "gain" (or sensitivity) of the unit, but again all echoes above the threshold are recorded at one intensity, and echoes below the threshold are not recorded at all. With gray scale units, echoes of many differing intensities are recorded, with stronger echoes appearing darker in proportion to their intensity. Thus, with no need to change the gain, fluid-filled structures can easily be differentiated from solid structures. In addition, the echographic characteristics of various solid organs often clearly differentiate the parenchyma of one from another.

Gray scale has been especially useful in evaluating the pancreas and the internal structure of the liver as well as in obstetric applications. The following cases include both bistable echograms and pictures obtained on a gray scale unit, so you can judge for yourself.

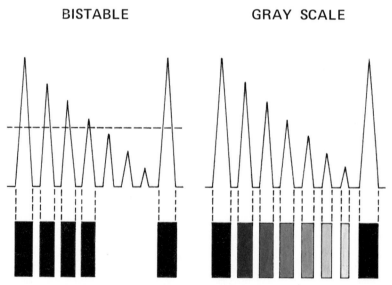

BISTABLE   GRAY SCALE

Fig. 1–9. **Diagram. Bistable and gray scale recordings. Note that echoes weaker than the threshold (dotted line) are *not* recorded with the bistable unit. Echoes stronger than the threshold are recorded at a single intensity. The gray scale recording, on the other hand, allows differentiation of a range of intensities.**

SUMMARY

1. The ultrasound beam is partially reflected at an *interface* between two tissues of differing acoustic impedance. The degree of difference in acoustic impedance determines the strength of the returning echo.

2. Air, bone, and barium all act as barriers to the ultrasonic beam. Air is an absolute barrier, reflecting over 99 per cent of the beam. Bone is a relative barrier, reflecting about 36 per cent of the beam, but allowing some ultrasound to penetrate.

3. Solid organs and masses generally have many weak internal echoes.

4. Fluid-filled organs and masses usually have no internal echoes, even when the sensitivity of the machine is turned up very high ("high gain").

CHAPTER 2

ABDOMINAL SCANNING

In order to appreciate abnormal findings, the student should have solid grounding in the many variations of normal that may be found in abdominal echograms. For convenience, all supine transverse sections in this book are marked by their relationship to the umbilicus. Sections cephalad to the umbilicus are designated positive sections, and those caudad are designated negative (e.g., a section designated U+4 was obtained 4 cm. cephalad to the umbilicus). If the umbilicus has been surgically removed, sections are related to the distance from the xiphoid process. Prone sections are related to the iliac crest. Longitudinal sections are related to their distance in centimeters from the midline of the body (e.g., a section designated R3 was obtained 3 cm. to the *right* of midline. A section designated L6 was obtained 6 cm. to the *left* of midline.)

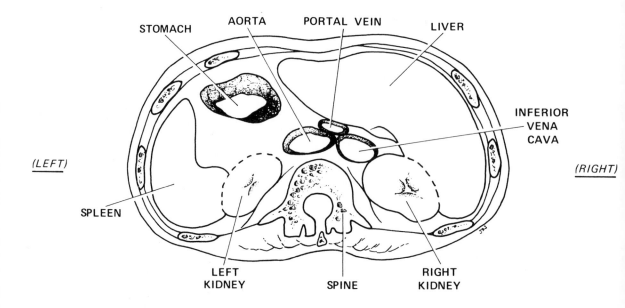

Fig. 2–1A. Transverse Supine. U+14

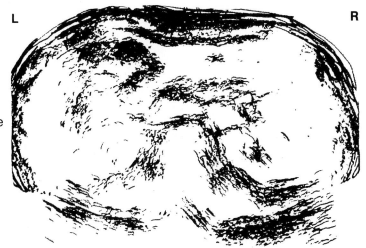

Fig. 2–1B. Bistable U+14 Supine

Figure 2–1B is a transverse supine section obtained on the bistable unit at U+14, and Figure 2–1A is a line drawing of this section. Figure 2–1C is the corresponding gray scale picture. Note the incomplete visualization of the left kidney on both scans: the anterior surface has been obscured by overlying stomach gas. At this level, the kidneys lie immediately lateral to the vertebral body. The spleen-kidney and liver-kidney interfaces are not completely defined, probably because at a level this cephalad the interfaces between the kidney and adjacent organs are oblique to the transducer and thus do not return strong echoes. *The more perpendicular an interface is to the transducer, the stronger will be the echoes returned.*

The aorta and inferior vena cava are clearly delineated. These pictures were obtained with the patient in end-inspiraton, a technique that produces distention of the inferior vena cava, allowing better visualization. On the gray scale study, the portal vein is also outlined. This is not seen as well on the bistable picture. The liver and spleen are of normal

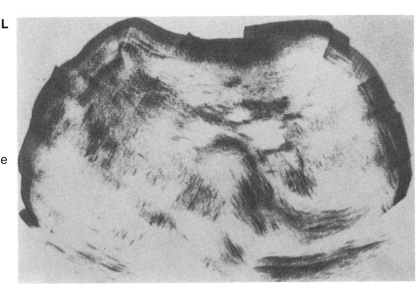

Fig. 2–1C.

Gray scale U+14 Supine

size. The stomach is represented by a dense semicircular collection of echoes returned from the area where the ultrasonic beam contacted the gas within the stomach fundus. A strong interface like this produces a dense collection of echoes, and acts as a barrier to further penetration of the beam.

Figures 2–2B and 2–2C are transverse supine sections of the abdomen at U+8, and Figure 2–2A is a line drawing of the section. At this level, the kidneys are separated from the vertebral body by the psoas muscles.

On the bistable study, why are the outlines of the gallbladder, right kidney, and posterior body wall somewhat darker than similar structures on the left? Look closely and you will see a similar dark area on the anterior body wall on the right. The technologist held the transducer on this spot for a while and "worked it over," producing a section of darker echoes as the transducer was directed several times over the same area.

On the gray scale study, you can see multiple fine gray echoes in the liver parenchyma. The renal parenchyma, on the other hand, is more lucent. Within the kidneys multiple strong central echoes represent echoes from the renal collecting system. The gallbladder is completely sonolucent (as befits a cystic structure), and stands out sharply from the liver parenchyma. Compare this with the gallbladder and liver parenchyma on the bistable study. The vena cava shows up well medial to the gallbladder. The aorta was not well outlined on this study.

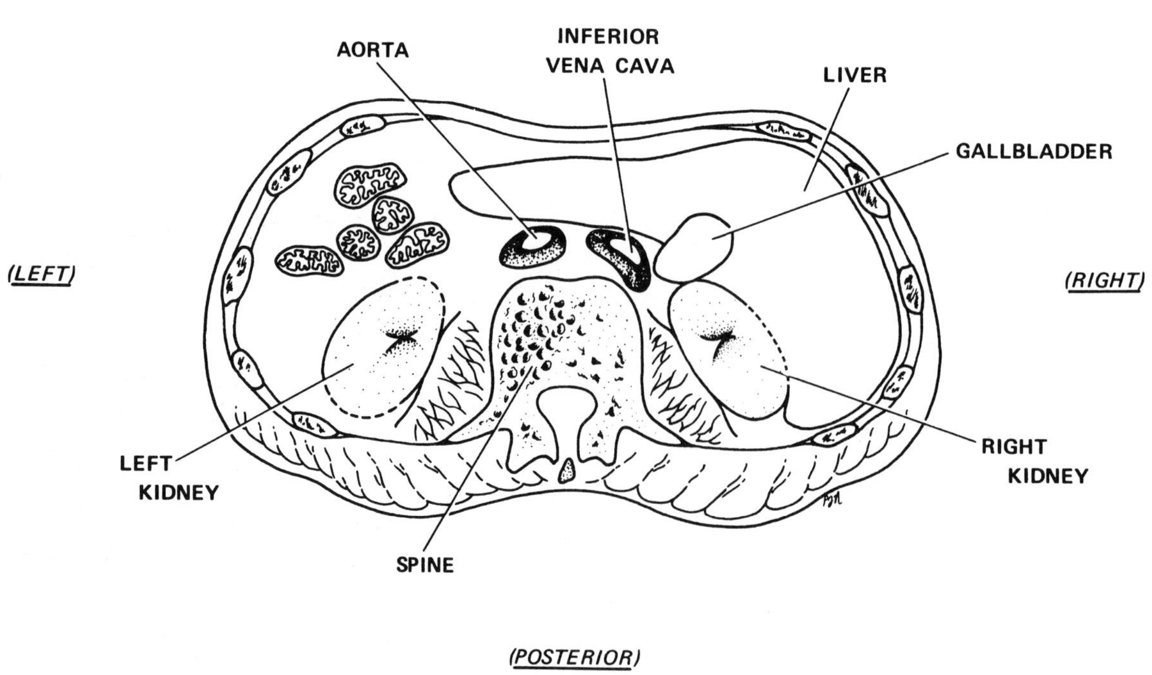

(ANTERIOR)

AORTA

INFERIOR VENA CAVA

LIVER

GALLBLADDER

(LEFT)

(RIGHT)

LEFT KIDNEY

RIGHT KIDNEY

SPINE

(POSTERIOR)

Fig. 2–2A. Transverse Supine U+8

L R

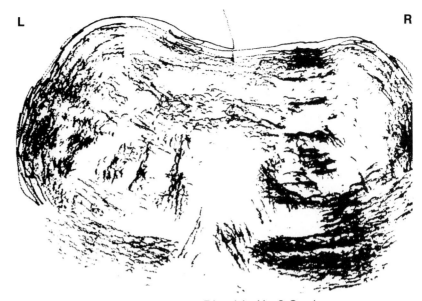

Fig. 2–2B. Bistable U+8 Supine

In this patient, why don't we see the left kidney as well on the gray scale as on the bistable study? Well, we brought the patient back for his gray scale study on another date, at which time the splenic flexure of his colon was filled with gas. This effectively impeded transmission of the ultrasound beam into the left upper quadrant, so that the left kidney could not be outlined. Frequently gas in the stomach will have the same effect. The patient must then be turned into the prone position for satisfactory examination of the kidneys.

L R

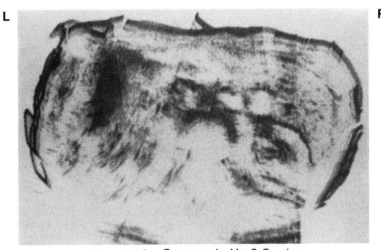

Fig. 2–2C. Gray scale U+8 Supine

Figures 2–3B and 2–3C are longitudinal supine sections approximately 6 cm. to the right of the midline (R6). Figure 2–3A is a line drawing of the section. Note the relationship of the gallbladder to the right kidney on these studies. Compare the relationship between these two organs on the transverse studies (Figs. 2–2B and 2–2C). On the longitudinal studies, the tip of the gallbladder is not sharply defined, owing to reverberations from nearby gas-filled bowel. Notice again how sonolucent the gallbladder appears when compared to the liver on the gray scale study. The right renal collecting system is seen on both studies, but the renal outlines are more clearly delineated on the gray scale picture.

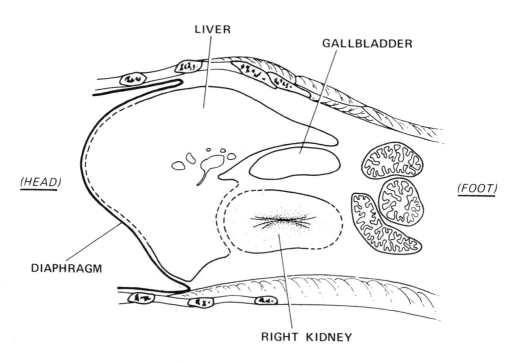

(ANTERIOR)

LIVER

GALLBLADDER

(HEAD)

(FOOT)

DIAPHRAGM

RIGHT KIDNEY

(POSTERIOR)

Fig. 2–3A. Longitudinal R 6 supine

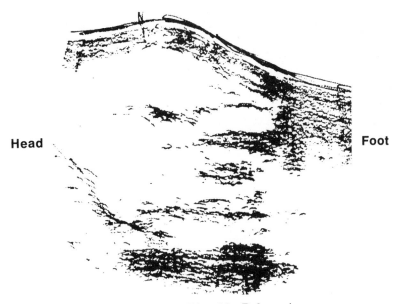

Head   **Foot**

Fig. 2–3B. Bistable R 6 supine

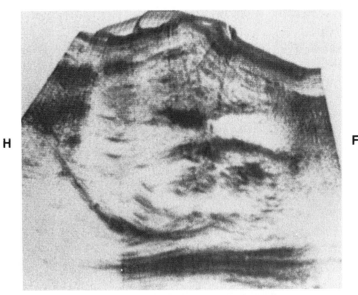

H   **F**

Fig. 2–3C. Gray scale R 6 supine

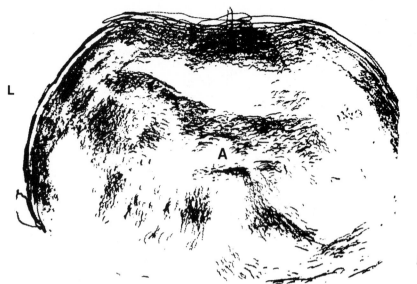

Fig. 2–4A. **Patient A**

FOUR DIFFERENT PATIENTS

All four of these transverse supine sections were obtained at a level approximately 14 cm. cephalad to the umbilicus (U+14). Study these echograms systematically. First find the vertebral body and the aorta (A), anterior to it and slightly to the left. Most students don't realize how far anterior the vertebral body extends in the average individual. Note that the aorta lies almost at the midpoint between the anterior and posterior body walls. Compare the shape of the liver, especially the left lobe, in each of these patients. Can you see the fissure between the right and left lobes of the liver in any of these patients? Which one? How far anterior is the tip of the spleen in comparison to the anterior wall of the aorta? One of the patients has an enlarged spleen. Which one? Are the kidneys seen well on all these pictures? How might you change the patient's position to improve renal visualization?

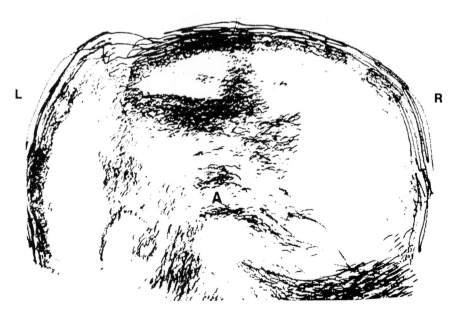

Fig. 2–4B. **Patient B**

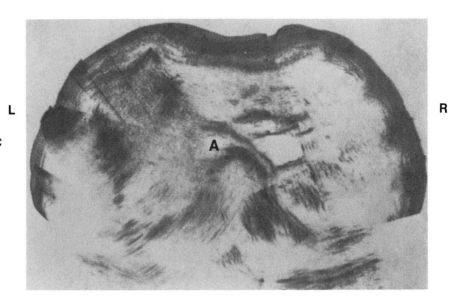

L   R

Fig. 2-4C. **Patient C**

A

ANSWERS

The shape and thickness of the left lobe of the liver is highly variable in normal people. The fissure between the right and left lobe of the liver is best seen in patient *B*. Patient *B* also has an enlarged spleen. Its tip extends almost to the anterior abdominal wall. A normal splenic tip rarely extends more than 1 cm. anterior to the anterior wall of the aorta. The left kidney can be seen on patients *A*, *B*, and *C*; the right kidney on patients *B* and *C*. For a better view of the kidneys, the patient must be examined in the prone position. In patient *D*, the scan was done at a level slightly too far cephalad to include the kidneys.

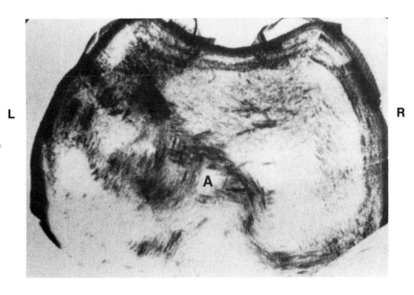

L   R

Fig. 2-4D. **Patient D**

A

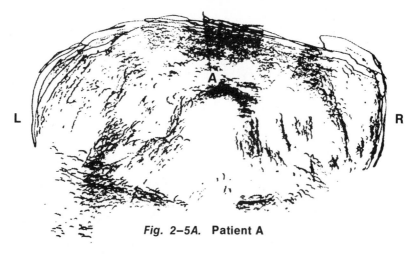

Fig. 2–5A. **Patient A**

FOUR MORE SUPINE STUDIES

In this next group of patients observe the general body outline. What does it tell you about the level at which the study was obtained? Notice that the aorta (A) is in the anterior *third* of the abdomen in patient A. This is commonly seen in sections obtained more inferiorly on thin patients. The aorta can be seen in all four of these patients, represented as an echo-free circular structure just anterior to the vertebral body in the midline or slightly to the left. In some patients (A and C) the aortic walls are not well outlined. This is partly a function of the examiner's technique. If the aorta were the primary area of interest in any of these patients, the examiner would have taken special care to outline it completely, probably at the expense of "overwriting" another area. That is, sometimes in order to see one organ well, the examiner must pass the transducer too many times over another structure, causing excessive recording of echoes from the latter area. This problem is largely obviated with gray scale units.

Note the better visualization of the kidneys (particularly the right kidney) in more caudad sections (patients A and D). The left kidney is obscured by overlying intestinal gas in patient A. In patients B and C, the sections were obtained at levels cephalad to the kidneys. What is the spherical left upper quadrant mass in patient C? Is it fluid filled or solid?

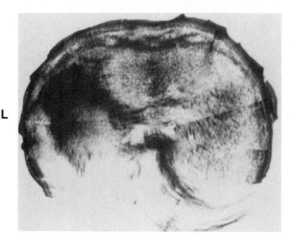

Fig. 2–5B. **Patient B**

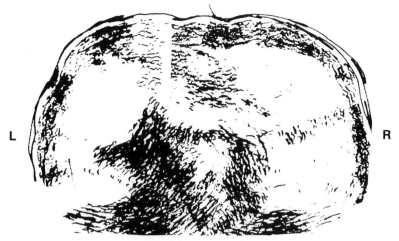

Fig. 2–5C. Patient C

ANSWERS

In most people, the AP diameter is less near the level of the umbilicus than it is in more cephalad sections. Thus, in patients *A* and *D*, the sections were obtained at a level well caudad to the body of the liver, cutting across the mid-portion of the kidneys. The liver tip is still visible in patient *D*, however, lying just to the right of the right kidney, and extending anteriorly. The spherical fluid-filled mass in the left upper quadrant of patient *C* represents the fluid-filled fundus of the stomach in a patient with gastric outlet obstruction. How can you tell that the mass is fluid rather than solid? Well, there are no internal echoes (and this was also true at high gain), the border farthest from the transducer is sharp, and there is high through transmission; these three characteristics indicate a very homogeneous mass, most likely fluid. When the picture was repeated with high gain (not shown), the liver filled in with echoes, whereas the fluid-filled stomach remained echo free, another clue to its homogeneous internal nature.

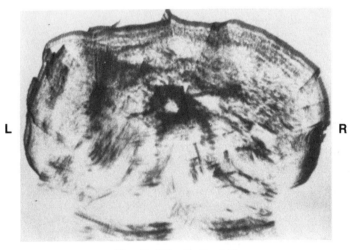

Fig. 2–5D. Patient D

GREAT VESSELS REVEALED

On the longitudinal view, the aorta and inferior vena cava can be clearly distinguished. Figure 2–6*A* shows a longitudinal section of the aorta obtained 1 cm. to the left of midline. Figure 2–6*B* shows a similar longitudinal section of the inferior vena cava obtained 1 cm. to the right of midline. This latter study was performed at end-inspiration, to produce maximum distention of the vessel. To provide an anatomic marker, the transducer was lifted from the abdomen at the level of the umbilicus.

Look at the course the two vessels take. The inferior vena cava is horizontal, moving slightly anteriorly at the level of the diaphragm in order to enter the right atrium. The aorta, on the other hand, moves more posteriorly as it approaches the diaphragm. These differing courses are easy to remember if you think of the position of the two vessels on the lateral chest film: the descending aorta lies far posterior, near the diaphragm, whereas the inferior vena cava lies midway between the anterior and posterior chest walls.

The round sonolucent structure just anterior to the inferior vena cava is the portal vein. In this normal patient, the portal vein, like the inferior vena cava, is also well distended at end-inspiration.

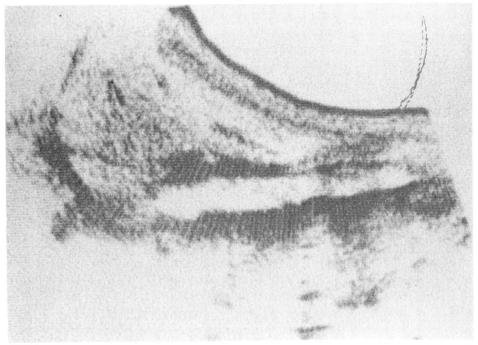

H   *Fig. 2–6A.* *Aorta.*   F

H   *Fig. 2–6B.* *Inferior vena cava.*   F

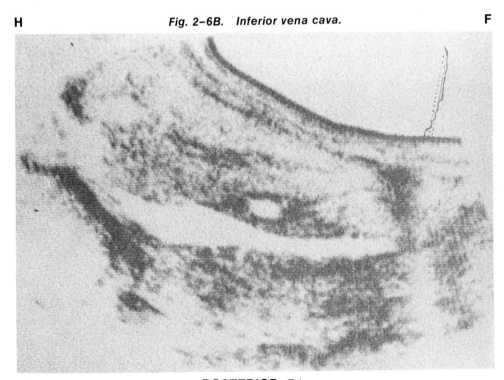

POSTERIOR R1

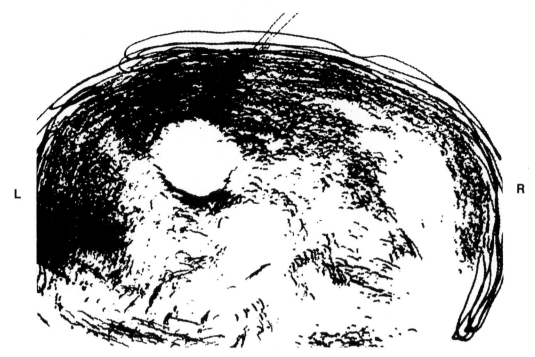

Fig. 2–7A. Transverse U+2 Supine

The aorta in Figure 2–7*A* is unusually large and far to the left. A longitudinal section over the vessel (Fig. 2–7*B*) more clearly delineates the area of aneurysmal dilatation (A). Note the longitudinal section of the left lobe of the liver (L) on the left-hand (cephalad) portion of the picture.

Any diameter of the aorta exceeding 3 cm. is, by definition, aneurysmal. In a patient with an asymptomatic aneurysm less than 5 cm. in diameter, ultrasound may be used to follow the patient at 3-to-6-month intervals. If the size and shape of the aneurysm are stable and the patient remains asymptomatic, surgery may be avoided.

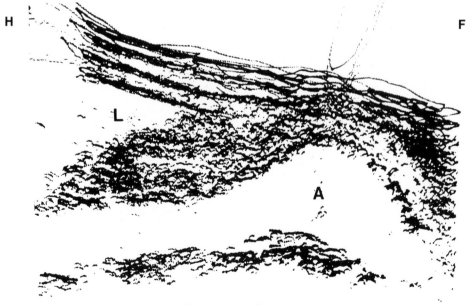

Fig. 2–7B. Supine L3

PROBLEM

This ultrasonic cross-section (Fig. 2–8A) was performed at a level 6 cm. above the umbilicus. Do you see the posterior part of the patient's body? The vertebral body? Is the beam penetrating well? What are two possible explanations for this phenomenon?

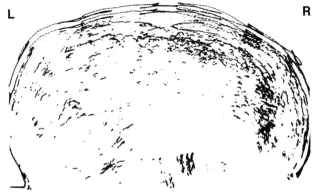

L R

Fig. 2–8A. Supine U+6

ANSWER

Figure 2–8B is a study done on the same patient two days later. Now the back and internal structures are easily seen, owing to satisfactory penetration of the ultrasonic beam. The previous study was of poor technical quality because the patient had just had an upper GI series, and the barium-filled gut impeded beam penetration. A similar problem would be encountered in a patient with many gas-filled bowel loops.

U+6

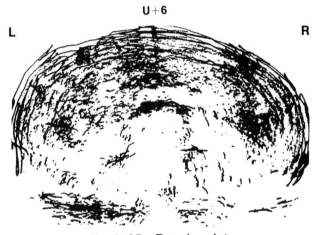

L R

Fig. 2–8B. Two days later

> SOUND ADVICE: Small amounts of air trapped between the transducer and the skin surface may also interfere with beam transmission. For this reason, a contact medium such as mineral oil or bubble-free gel is applied to the patient's skin before scanning. This allows satisfactory contact between transducer and skin, with no air interference.

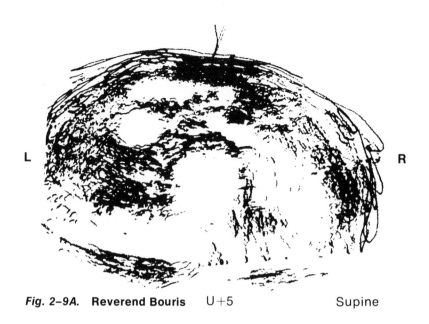

Fig. 2–9A. **Reverend Bouris** U+5   Supine

THREE PATIENTS WHO PRESENT WITH WEIGHT LOSS

Ken Bouris, a 35-year-old preacher, was well until three or four months ago, when he began to notice increasing fatigue. Despite gourmet tastes, he has lost 20 pounds in three months. Physical examination is entirely normal.

Helen Flegenheimer, 51, a writer specializing in political whitewash reminiscences, has noted a 15 pound weight loss over the last two months, which she attributes to loss of interest in eating. She appears exhausted, but her physical examination is normal.

U+8   Supine

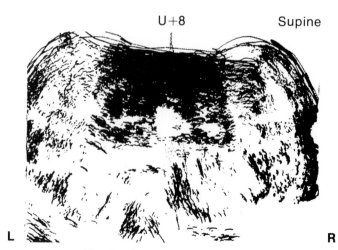

Fig. 2–10A. **Mrs. Flegenheimer**

U+1   Supine

L 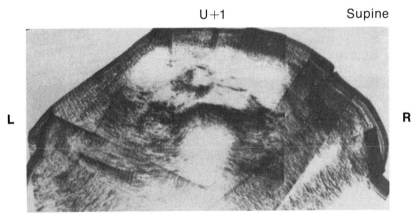 R

Fig. 2–11A. **Mr. Yankey**

Dan Yankey, a 56-year-old historian, has been increasingly irritable in the last two months. He attributes this to the frustration engendered by the encroachment of teaching responsibilities on his research time. But his 18 pound weight loss is hard to ignore. Mr. Yankey appears tense, irritable, and chronically ill.

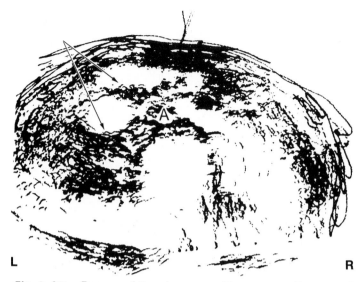

Reverend Bouris's transverse echogram (Fig. 2–9B) reveals several sonolucent masses (arrows) in the midabdomen, extending slightly to the left. On repeat palpation of the abdomen, these masses still could not be felt. Although the masses are sonolucent even at high gain, there is no evidence of high through transmission, indicating that they may be homogeneous *solid* structures.

L   R

Fig. 2–9B. **Reverend Bouris**   Transverse Repeated

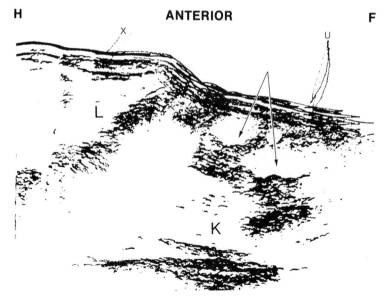

H   ANTERIOR   F

On the longitudinal study (Fig. 2–9C) the masses (arrows) are again well delineated, the more cephalad one lying anterior to the left kidney (K). To provide anatomic markers, the transducer was lifted from the body at the level of the xiphoid (X) and again at the level of the umbilicus (U). This convention is used on most of the longitudinal studies in this chapter.

Fig. 2–9C. **Reverend Bouris**   **L6**

GALLIUM SCAN SUPERIMPOSED ON A DIAGRAM OF THE SKELETON

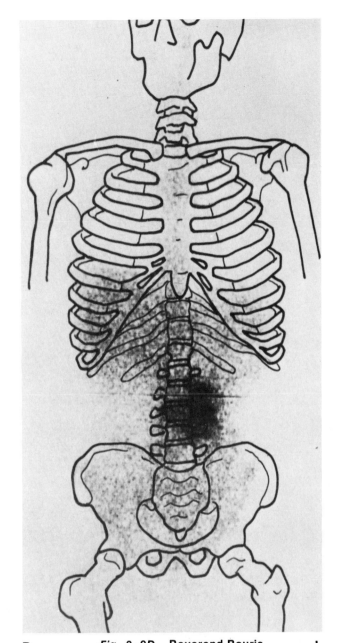

R   *Fig. 2–9D.* **Reverend Bouris**   L

Courtesy of Dr. Naomi Alazraki

Upper and lower GI series and IVP (not shown) were entirely normal. The patient was then scanned with Gallium^{67} (^{67}Ga), an isotope that concentrates in certain tumors and also in abscesses. There was uptake of the isotope in the region of the masses (Fig. 2–9D). At surgery, it was revealed that *Reverend Bouris* had Hodgkin's disease involving the mesentery. (This is why the masses couldn't be demonstrated with barium or palpated. They just moved away from the palpating hand.)

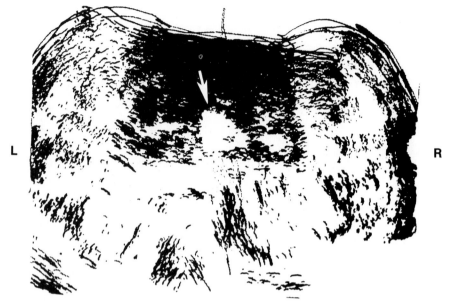

Fig. 2–10B. **Mrs. Flegenheimer** Transverse Repeated

Mrs. Flegenheimer has a suspicious-looking mass in her midabdomen (arrow), just anterior to the region of the inferior vena cava (the cava itself is not clearly outlined). A slightly smaller mass is seen just to the right. There was no evidence of high through transmission, and several echoes are seen within. The dark echoes across the anterior midabdomen are due to the fact that the technologist "worked over" the area, repeatedly passing the transducer across it in an effort to improve visualization of the mass. The pancreas lies in this location, and this appearance is highly suggestive of a pancreatic mass.

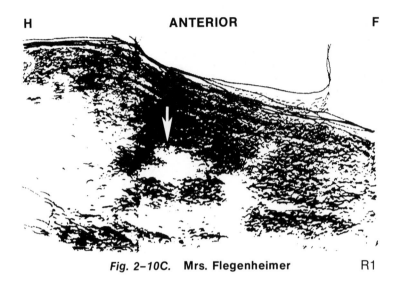

H **ANTERIOR** **F**

Fig. 2–10C. **Mrs. Flegenheimer** R1

The mass (arrow) can also be seen on longitudinal scan (Fig. 2–10C). Hypotonic duodenogram (not shown) and abdominal angiogram (including selective injections for pancreatic study) were reported normal. At surgery, there was a large carcinoma in the pancreatic body, with metastases in lymph nodes near the pancreatic head. These findings account for the *two* masses seen on the echogram. The hypotonic duodenogram was normal because the pancreatic head itself was not involved.

L   R

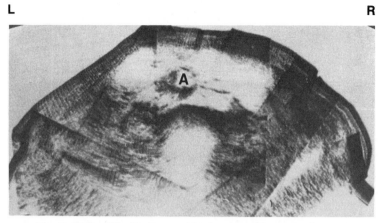

Fig. 2-11B. **Mr. Yankey**   U+1   Repeated

Mr. Yankey's aorta (A) is surrounded and displaced anteriorly away from the vertebral body by an irregular sonolucent mass. A scan performed 2 cm. *caudad* to the umbilicus (Fig. 2-11C) shows the iliac vessels also displaced anteriorly and surrounded by this mass.

L   R

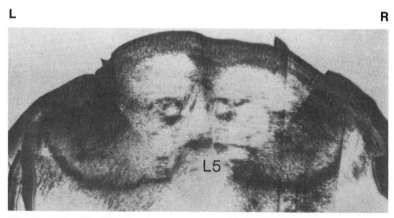

Fig. 2-11C. **Mr. Yankey**   U-2

IVP (Fig. 2–11D) shows slight lateral deviation of the left ureter. Note the normal kinking of the right ureter.

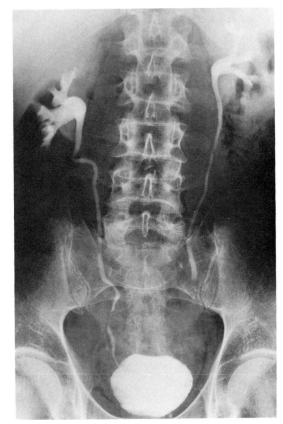

R   *Fig. 2–11D.* **Mr. Yankey** IVP   L

R   **L**

On ⁶⁷Ga scan (Fig. 2–11E), uptake extends along the entire periaortic region and into the right pelvis. Biopsy revealed reticulum cell sarcoma.

Fig. 2–11E. **Mr. Yankey**
GALLIUM STUDY

Courtesy of Dr. Naomi Alazraki

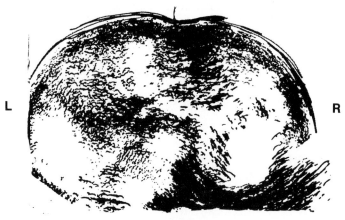

Fig. 2–12A. **Ms. Cadwallader**   U+17

THREE PATIENTS WITH SURGERY OR OTHER TRAUMA

Linda Cadwallader, the 27-year-old junior Congresswoman from the 17th District, sped too rapidly around a curve while commuting to work. She was thrown from her motorcycle and sustained multiple fractures. In addition, she complains of right upper quadrant pain. Her hematocrit on admission was 42. Now, six hours later, it is 35.

Clay Potter, a 22-year-old artisan, also had a recent motorcycle accident which necessitated removal of his spleen. Now, five weeks after surgery, he re-enters the hospital complaining of left upper quadrant pain and inability to take a deep breath because of the pain. T 100.2° F, WBC 16000/mm³.

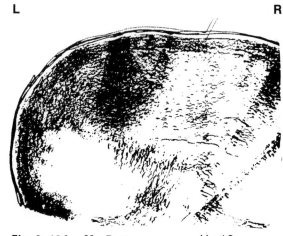

Fig. 2–13A. **Mr. Potter**   U+16

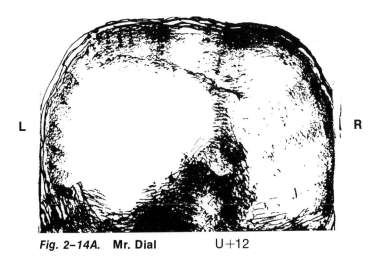

Fig. 2–14A. **Mr. Dial**   U+12

Four months ago **Crocker Dial,** 38, Florida land speculator, had his spleen removed. The surgery was performed in another country, and Crocker is not certain why it was done. Recently he has noticed some fatigue, and has difficulty buttoning up his pants. Physical examination reveals a prominent abdomen with no palpable masses or organomegaly.

ANSWERS

L
R

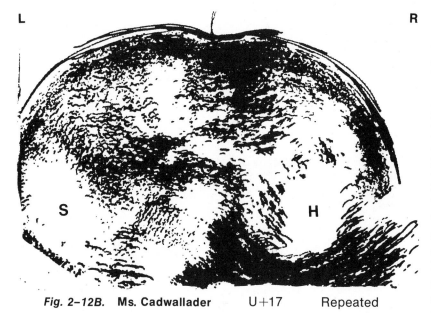

Fig. 2–12B. **Ms. Cadwallader**   U+17   Repeated

The echogram on *Ms. Cadwallader* (Fig. 2–12B) shows a large sonolucent area (H) posterolateral to the liver, with high through transmission beyond. Much of the normal liver parenchyma fills in with echoes due to the high gain which was used. Note that the spleen (S), an organ composed mostly of blood, is also relatively sonolucent. On gray scale studies, there are usually fine light-gray echoes in the spleen. These are below the threshold of resolution on this bistable study.

L
U+13
R

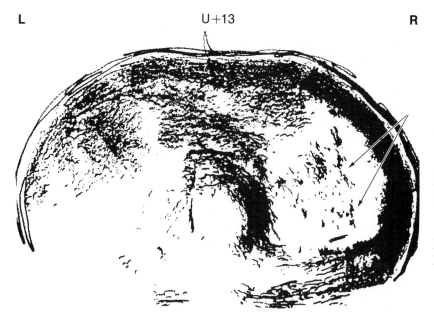

Fig. 2–12C. **Ms. Cadwallader**

In a section obtained at U + 13, somewhat more caudad (Fig. 2–12C), the sonolucent area is again seen. In this latter section, the sonolucent area extends lateral to the liver, pushing the liver medially (arrows indicate the medially displaced lateral border of the liver).

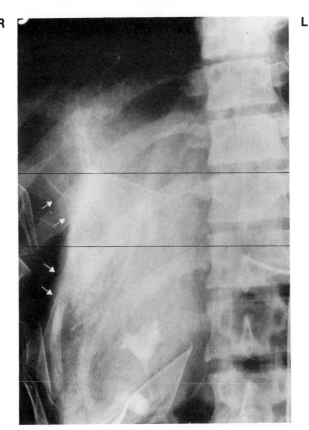

Fig. 2–12D. **Ms. Cadwallader**

Arteriogram (hepatogram phase). The horizontal lines indicate the levels of the two echographic sections.

Arteriogram (Fig. 2–12D) confirmed medial displacement of the liver by an avascular mass lying laterally. The posterior extent of the mass was not evaluated with angiography, as all films were obtained in the AP projection. On this radiograph, obtained during the parenchymal phase of the arteriogram, the medially displaced liver appears dense, owing to staining by contrast, some of which is already seen in the renal collecting system. Note the avascular area (with overlying dressings) lateral to the liver edge (arrows). The patient did well after drainage of her hepatic subcapsular hematoma.

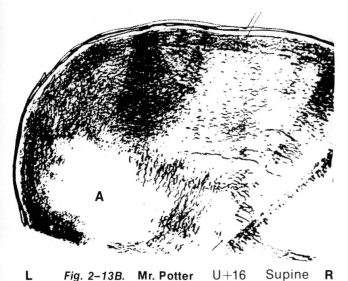

Ultrasound examination of *Mr. Potter* (Fig. 2–13*B*) was somewhat impaired by the presence of increased intestinal gas (not unusual in a patient with abdominal pain). However, the echogram of the left upper quadrant revealed a large, well-defined, sonolucent mass (A). The shape of the mass is a little more rounded than is usually seen with the spleen. (Compare Figure 2–12*B*). Anyway, this patient has had a splenectomy.

L   *Fig. 2–13B.* **Mr. Potter**   U+16   Supine   **R**

When the patient was turned to the *prone* position (Fig. 2–13*C*), it became more apparent that there was high through transmission beyond the mass. Occasional small internal echoes within the mass were also noted. This type of echogram, having the characteristics of both fluid (largely sonolucent, high through transmission), and solid (occasional internal echoes) masses, may be seen in two types of lesions: fluid-filled masses with some internal debris or septae, producing internal echoes (e.g., abscess); and in necrotic tumors.

R   **L**

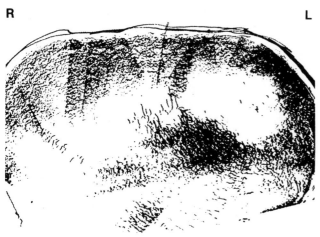

Note that in the prone position, the section is viewed as if seen from the patient's head. For this reason, the positions of the left and right sides of the body are reversed when compared with the supine scan.

Fig. 2–13C. **Mr. Potter**   IC+16   Prone

R   L

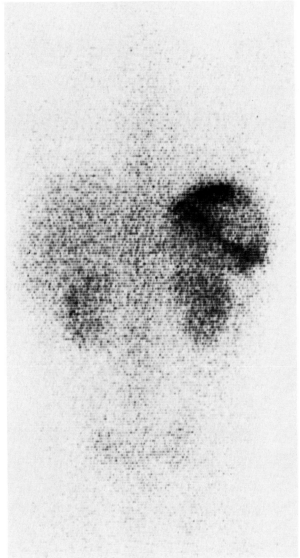

Fig. 2-13D. Gallium study Mr. Potter

Courtesy of Dr. Naomi Alazraki.

In view of the patient's history, abscess was the most likely diagnosis. ^{67}Ga scan (Fig. 2-13D) showed uptake of isotope in the periphery of the lesion, confirming the presence of a large subdiaphragmatic abscess. At surgery, 500 cc. of purulent material was drained. Incidentally, this is the first ^{67}Ga scan in this book that does not have a superimposed skeleton. By identifying the uptake in the vertical strip of the spine and also in the pelvic bones, you can mentally superimpose the skeleton yourself.

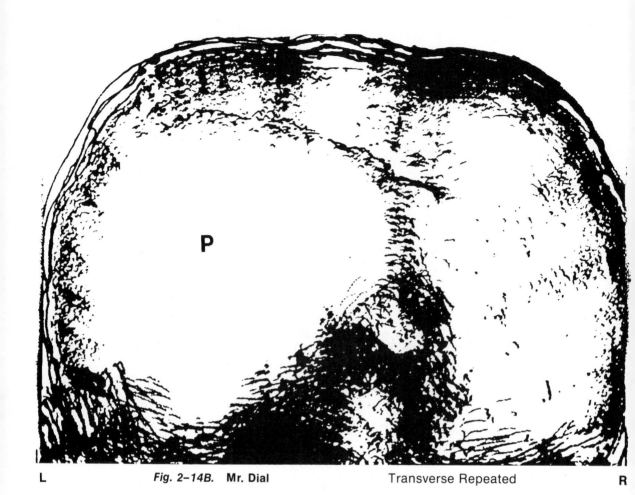

L   *Fig. 2–14B.* **Mr. Dial**   Transverse Repeated   R

There's no doubt that *Mr. Dial* has a *large* fluid-filled mass (P) in his left upper quadrant. Upper GI series (Fig. 2–14C) confirms the presence of a mass displacing the stomach medially and inferiorly. Laparotomy revealed it to be a huge pancreatic pseudocyst. It probably originated on a traumatic basis, related to the patient's previous surgery.

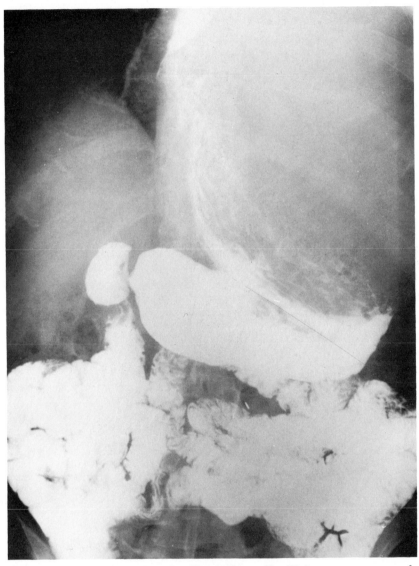

Fig. 2–14C. **Upper GI** **Mr. Dial**

R   L

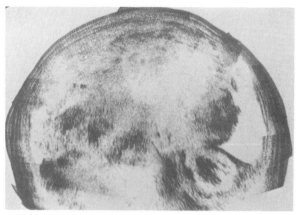

L *Fig. 2–15A.* **Ms. Reardon** U+6 R

THREE PATIENTS WITH INCREASED ABDOMINAL GIRTH

Salonica Reardon, a society matron of 50, formerly a tidy size 12, has been buying size 18 dresses ("for the mature figure") for the past four months. She doesn't think she could be pregnant, but is at a loss to explain her abdominal protuberance. Physical examination shows no evidence of abdominal mass. Shifting dullness is evident, however. And Ms. Reardon drinks a little. . . .

Cherie Freely, a 37-year-old stripper, has also noticed gradually increasing abdominal girth. This morning she was fired, and has concluded that it's time to see the doctor. Physical examination reveals a large, poorly defined mass which extends into the pelvis. It seems to be separate from the uterus.

L R

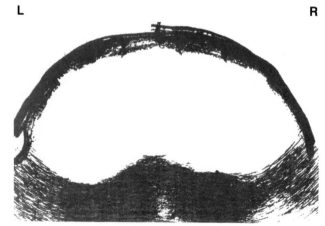

Fig. 2–16A. **Cherie** U–2

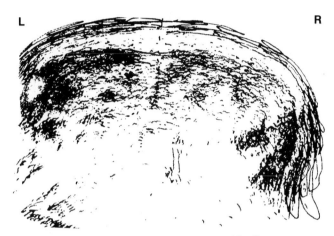

Fig. 2–17A. **Mrs. Waite** U+2

Carrie Waite, age 53, a housewife, has noted increasing abdominal girth, particularly prominent in the past year. Physical examination reveals an obese woman with no definite abdominal masses or fluid, however, palpation is difficult, owing to the patient's obesity. BP 170/100 mm Hg.

ANSWERS

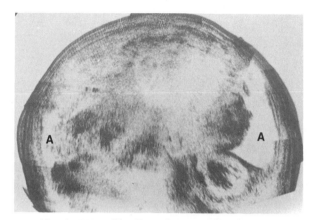

L   *Fig. 2–15B.*   **Ms. Reardon**   Transverse   R
Repeated

Ms. Reardon has ascites. Her echogram (Fig. 2–15B) shows a large collection of fluid (A) in both flanks, particularly on the right. There is poor definition of the aorta, inferior vena cava, and vertebral body, due to interference from gasfilled loops of bowel floating anteriorly in the midabdomen.

This is also clearly seen in the plain film of the abdomen (Fig. 2–15C). Note how small and large bowel loops are displaced centrally. The flanks and pelvis have a generalized gray appearance on the radiograph, caused by large amounts of ascitic fluid in these areas.

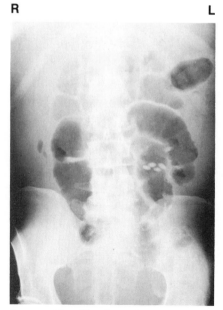

Fig. 2–15C.   **Ms. Reardon's plain film**

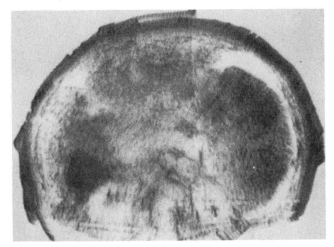

L   *Fig. 2–15D.* **Ms. Reardon**   U+10   R

An echogram obtained at a more cephalad level shows fluid lateral to the liver (L), displacing it medially. The liver has many dense internal echoes, due to the patient's cirrhosis.

On longitudinal scan (Fig. 2–15E), the liver tip (L) is surrounded by ascitic fluid, separating it from the kidney (K). Have you been wondering about those four ovoid densities on the abdominal film? Those are pills traveling through the intestines, still waiting to be absorbed.

H   F

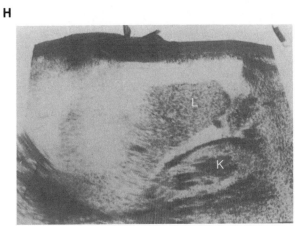

Fig. 2–15E. **Ms. Reardon**   R5

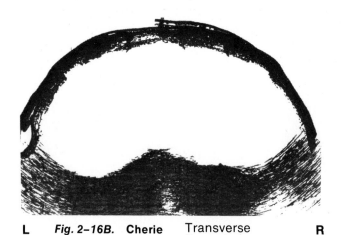

L   *Fig. 2–16B.* **Cherie**   Transverse   R
Repeated

Cherie's transverse echogram is a bit startling. Her entire abdominal cavity is occupied by a huge sonolucent mass with high through transmission.

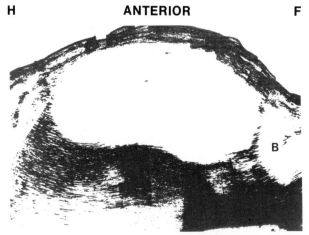

H   **ANTERIOR**   F

Fig. 2–16C. **Cherie**   Midline

Longitudinal study (Fig. 2–16C) shows that this mass extends from the pelvis almost to the liver. The bladder (B) is full, pushing the mass superiorly. At surgery, a giant ovarian cyst was removed.

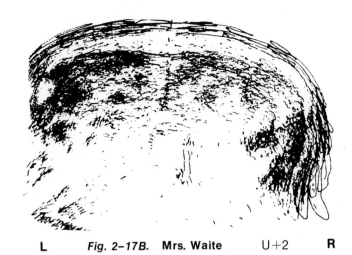

L   *Fig. 2–17B.*   **Mrs. Waite**   U+2   **R**

Echography on *Mrs. Waite* was somewhat unrewarding. The relatively sonolucent strip of tissue seen anteriorly represents fat. It can be seen even better on the longitudinal view (Fig. 2–17C). Also on the longitudinal study, note the triangular left lobe of the liver (L) and the aorta (A) lying beneath. There are no echoes beyond the aorta because the beam is blocked by the spine. The aorta is poorly seen just cephalad to the umbilical marker. Visualization in this region is impeded by gas-filled bowel. Obese patients are often poor subjects for echography.

ANTERIOR

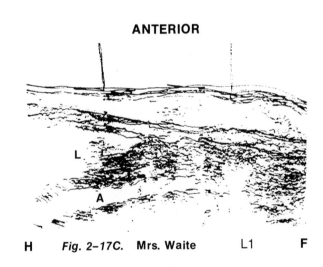

H   *Fig. 2–17C.*   **Mrs. Waite**   L1   **F**

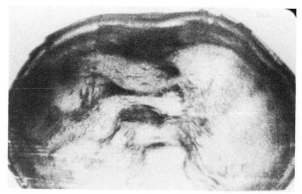

L   *Fig. 2–18A.* **Donna**   U+8   R

Donna A. Mobile, a 35-year-old country and western singer, collapsed during a rehearsal, complaining of severe abdominal pain. Her epigastrium is tender but not rigid. Bowel sounds are decreased. Rectal and pelvic examinations are negative. T 99.2° F., WBC 13000/mm³, Amylase 2000 Somogyi units.

THREE PATIENTS WITH ABDOMINAL PAIN

Chuck Friendly, 43, recreational vehicle salesman, couldn't resist another helping of fried chicken at the company picnic. Two hours later he was in the Emergency Room, complaining of severe right upper quadrant pain and nausea. This has happened to Chuck before. Physical exam reveals an obese man in moderate distress with right upper quadrant tenderness and guarding. There were no palpable masses. T 99.8° F.

L   R

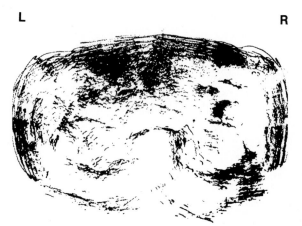

Fig. 2–19A. **Mr. Friendly**   U+7

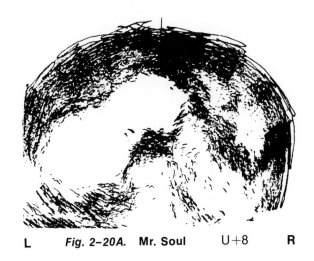

L   *Fig. 2–20A.*   **Mr. Soul**   U+8   **R**

Theodosius Soul, 66 years old, is a jazz musician. He complains of severe abdominal pain radiating to his back. The pain began approximately three days ago and is becoming gradually more severe. Physical exam reveals a pulsating tender midabdominal mass. Serial hematocrits are stable.

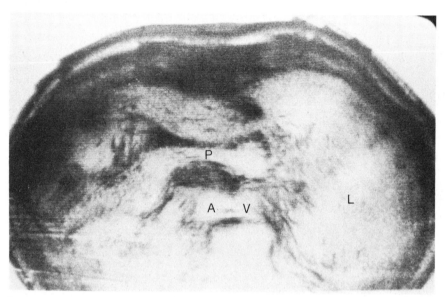

L   *Fig. 2–18B.* **Donna**   Transverse Repeated   **R**

Donna's echogram reveals a long, relatively sonolucent mass (P) lying just anterior to the great vessels (A,V). This appearance is characteristic of general-ized pancreatic edema. The upper GI series (not shown) on this patient ap-peared normal; however, the duodenal sweep did not fill well.

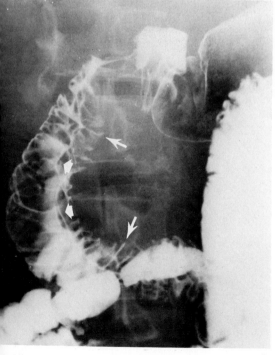

Glucagon was administered to induce duodenal relaxation, and more barium was given ("hypotonic duodenogram," Fig. 2–18C). Now you can see the scalloped im-pression on the medial portion of the duo-denal sweep (arrowheads), due to the en-larged pancreatic head. There is also an appearance of "spiculation" (arrows), caused by small streaks of barium trapped between edematous folds. All these find-ings are commonly seen with pancreatitis.

Fig. 2–18C. **Hypotonic duodenogram**

L

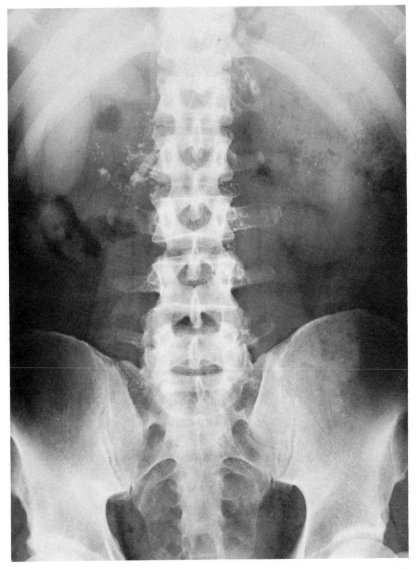

R   *Fig. 2–18D.*   Donna's plain film   L

Do you see the flecks of calcium extending obliquely across the midabdomen on *Donna's* plain film? They can also be faintly seen medial to the duodenal sweep on the hypotonic study. This finding of calcium in the pancreas is characteristic of chronic pancreatitis. Although *Donna* presented with an acute episode, further history taking revealed that she had had this problem before. The oval dense structure in the right upper quadrant on the plain film is a normal gallbladder, outlined by contrast material which this patient ingested the previous evening.

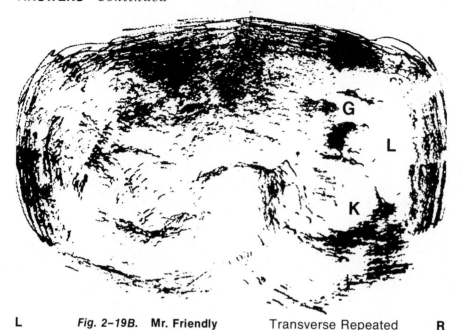

L   *Fig. 2–19B.* **Mr. Friendly**   Transverse Repeated   **R**

The transverse echogram on *Mr. Friendly* is entirely normal (Fig. 2–19B). Both kidneys (K) can be seen, just lateral to the psoas muscles. The aorta and vena cava are incompletely outlined, lying anterior to the spine. A small segment of liver (L) can also be seen. On the medial border of the liver is a sonolucent area (G) with sharp anterior and posterior borders and many echoes behind. This is a characteristic appearance of the gallbladder.

Longitudinal study of the same organ (Fig. 2–19C) showed a surprise. There was a collection of small echoes within (arrow). The diagnosis of gallstones was made on this study. Oral cholecystogram showed no visualization of the gallbladder, a common finding in acute cholecystitis. Two days later the surgeons removed a severely infected gallbladder containing multiple stones.

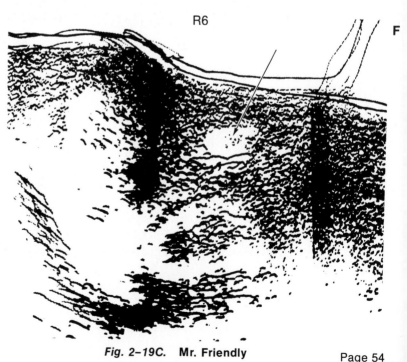

Fig. 2–19C. **Mr. Friendly**

STONED AGAIN

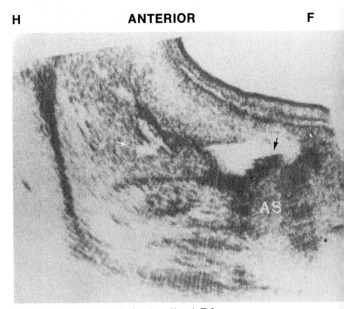

Fig. 2–19D.   Longitudinal R6

Figures 2–19D and 2–19E show longitudinal sections of the gallbladder on two patients with similar symptoms. In both patients, the dense echoes seen along the posterior wall of the gallbladder represent gallstones (arrow, Fig. 2–19D). Notice the decreased number of echoes immediately posterior to the stones on both pictures. This "acoustic shadow" (AS) occurs because the stones produce a strong interface, allowing little transmission of echoes beyond. In Figure 2–19D, can you identify the diaphragm, right kidney, and liver? The linear lucencies within the liver are venous branches.

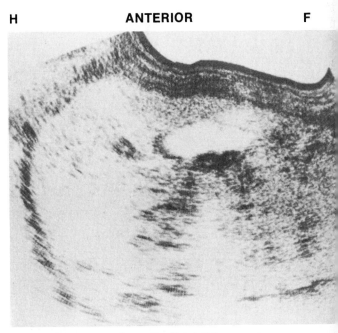

Fig. 2–19E.   Longitudinal R4

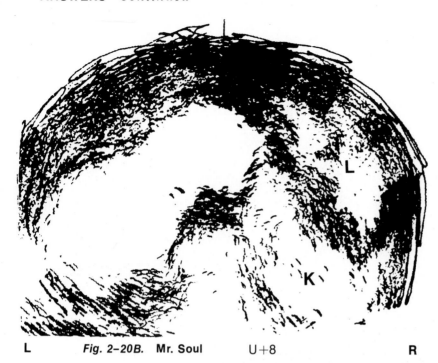

Mr. Soul's echogram (Fig. 2–20B) is clearly abnormal. A small portion of kidney (K) and liver (L) can be seen on the right. The remainder of the abdomen is filled with a bilobulated sonolucent mass showing high through transmission.

L   *Fig. 2–20B.* **Mr. Soul**   U+8   R

On the high gain study (Fig. 2–20C) there was partial separation of the two components, with the more posterior portion (H) containing some internal echoes. The longitudinal study (not shown) showed the more anterior mass (A) to represent a large aortic aneurysm.

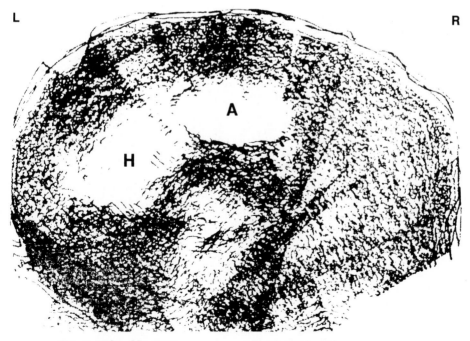

Fig. 2–20C. **Mr. Soul**   U+8 High gain

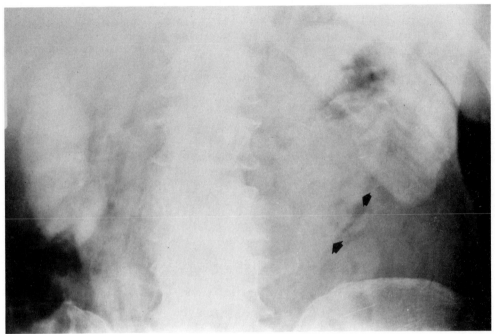

Fig. 2–20D. **Mr. Soul's IVP (nephrogram phase)**

On the nephrogram phase of the IVP (Fig. 2–20D), the left kidney is deviated laterally by the aneurysm (arrows). At surgery a massive, partially organized, left upper quadrant hematoma was found, which extended posteriorly from a small rupture in the aneurysm. This was the other part of the mass. Internal echoes are characteristically seen in organized thrombi.

Grey Fantome is a 32-year-old ghost writer who visits his family physician because he's "tired all the time." He appears pale, tired, and chronically ill. Physical examination reveals a left upper quadrant mass. T 99.6° F, WBC 25000/mm³.

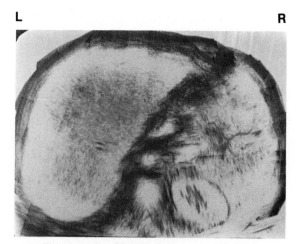

Fig. 2–21A. **Mr. Fantome** U+10

FOUR PATIENTS WITH AN ABDOMINAL MASS

L U+3 (close-up) R

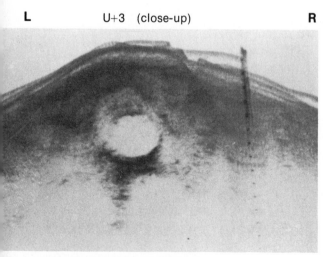

William Bligh, 73, retired sea captain (and owner of "The Lesser Breadfruit" Polynesian restaurant), comes to see you because he feels "something pulsing" in his abdomen. You feel it too, and request an abdominal echogram.

Fig. 2–22A. **Captain Bligh**

Duke Mantua, 39, former teenage gang leader (presently on parole), is hurriedly dropped off in the Emergency Room by some of his acquaintances. Duke smells of alcohol, and clutches his stomach, groaning. Physical exam reveals epigastric tenderness. There *may* be an epigastric mass; however, the patient is difficult to examine, and you are not certain of the finding.

L R

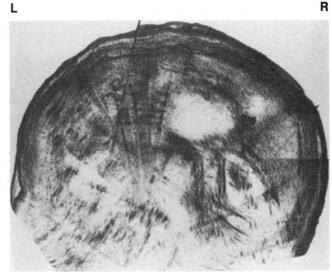

Fig. 2–23A. **Duke** U+8

Reginald Canting is a 46-year-old philosopher who was feeling perfectly well until he felt a rock-hard mass in his right midabdomen. This finding was confirmed by his physician, who found no additional abnormalities on physical examination. The patient was sent for an abdominal echogram even before results of blood work or urinalysis were available (honest!).

L R

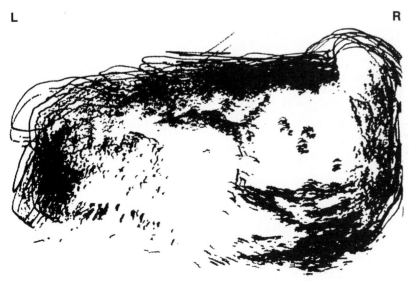

Fig. 2–24A. **Dr. Canting** U+4

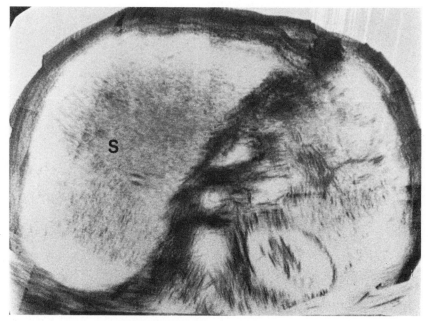

L   *Fig. 2–21B.* **Mr. Fantome**   Transverse Repeated   R

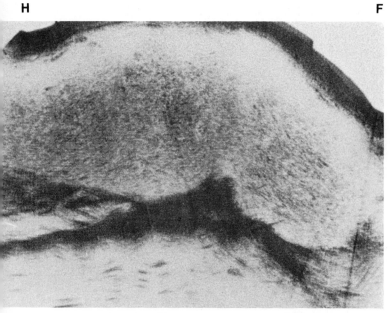

Fig. 2–21C. **Mr. Fantome**   L6

On first looking at *Mr. Fantome's* echogram (Fig. 2–21B) you may wonder (justifiably) if the patient has situs inversus. Actually, the left upper quadrant mass is a massively enlarged spleen (S). Figure 2–21C is a longitudinal view of the spleen.

On the plain film of the abdomen (Fig. 2–21D), the splenomegaly is also apparent. Further workup proved the diagnosis of chronic lymphocytic leukemia.

R   L

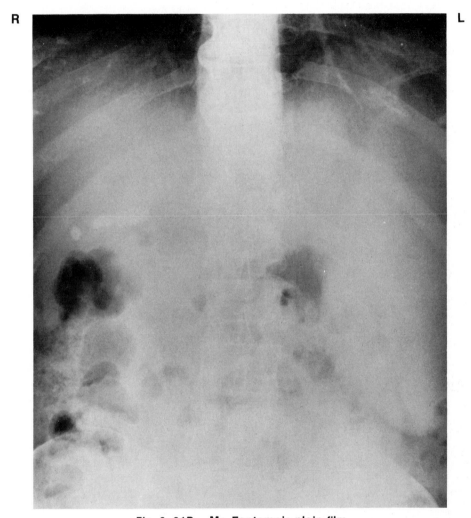

Fig. 2–21D.   **Mr. Fantome's plain film**

Incidentally, did you notice the linear collection of rounded densities in the right upper quadrant on this radiograph? If you thought they were gallstones, you're right again!

H   F

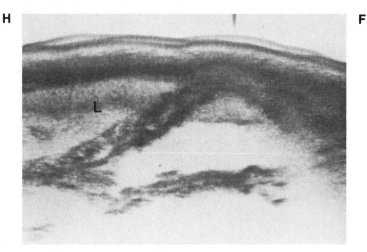

Fig. 2–22B.   **Captain Bligh**   L2

ANSWERS — *Continued*

R   L

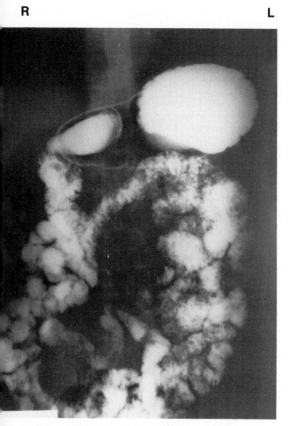

Captain Bligh's echograms (Figs. 2–22A and 2–22B) show aneurysmal dilatation of the abdominal aorta. Fine echoes anteriorly within the aneurysm represent thrombus. The aneurysm extends into the right iliac artery (echogram not shown). This iliac extension can be readily appreciated on the upper GI series (Fig. 2–22C), which was obtained to evaluate the patient's additional complaints of epigastric distress. Note the displacement of the small bowel by the aortic and right iliac aneurysms.

Fig. 2–22C.   **Captain Bligh**   UGI

L   R

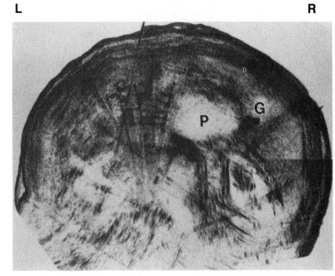

Echogram (Fig. 2–23B) confirms your suspicion of a mass (P) in *Duke's* abdomen. The mass is sonolucent, has high through transmission, and lies just medial to the liver and beneath the left lobe. (Hmm... that's the pancreatic area again.) Upper GI series (Fig. 2–23C) shows displacement of the stomach by the mass. The patient was treated medically for his pancreatitis, and was followed by ultrasound at weekly intervals. After six weeks, there was no change in the appearance of the mass. At surgery, a large pseudocyst was drained.

Fig. 2–23B. **Duke**   Transverse Repeated

R   L

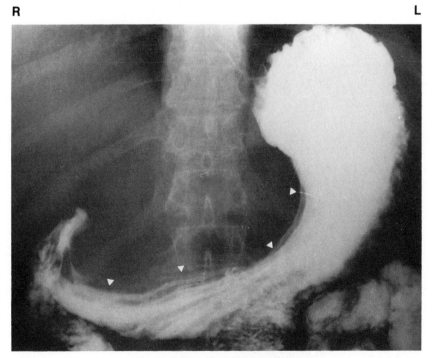

Fig. 2–23C. **Duke's stomach**

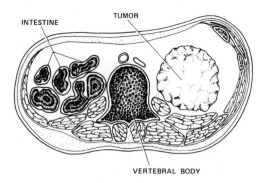

INTESTINE TUMOR

VERTEBRAL BODY

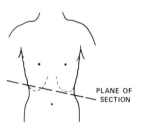

PLANE OF SECTION

Fig. 2–24B. **Diagram. Plane of section used to obtain echogram in Figure 2–24A. The section was inadvertently obtained in a slightly oblique plane. This explains the asymmetry of the body outline on the echogram.**

Dr. Canting's echogram (Fig. 2–24A) confirms the presence of a solid mass. Don't be confused by the apparent asymmetry of this patient's abdominal wall. The section was slightly oblique (Fig. 2–24B), so that on the right the transducer outlined the rise of the costal margin, whereas on the left, the transducer was still caudad to the ribs. On the longitudinal supine study (Fig. 2–24C), the mass (arrows) is seen just inferior to the liver (L).

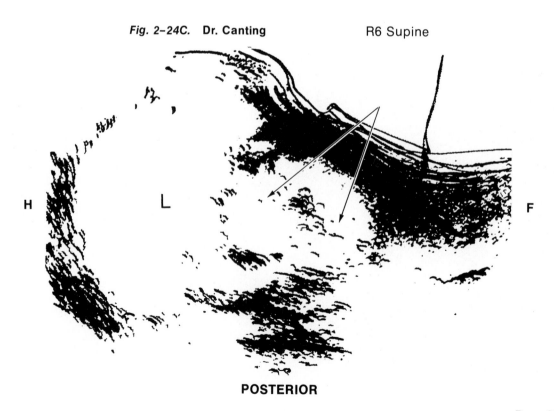

Fig. 2–24C. **Dr. Canting**   R6 Supine

H   L   F

POSTERIOR

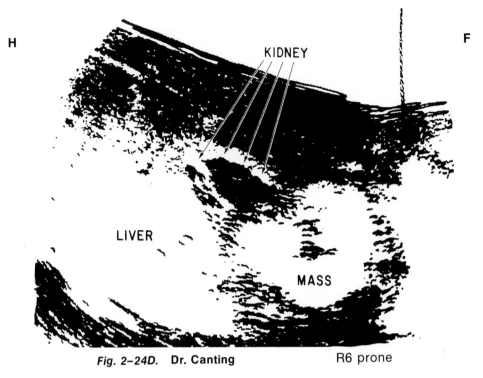

H

F

KIDNEY

LIVER

MASS

Fig. 2–24D. **Dr. Canting**   R6 prone

Right renal arteriogram

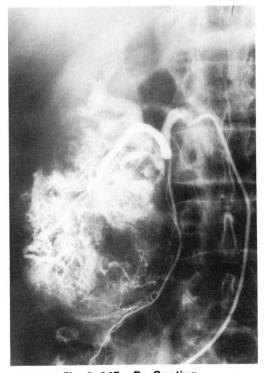

Fig. 2–24E. **Dr. Canting**

The right kidney could not be demonstrated on the supine examination, however, which made the sonographer suspicious. On the *prone* longitudinal study (Fig. 2–24D), the mass is clearly seen extending from the lower pole of the right kidney. IVP and angiogram (Fig. 2–24E) confirmed the diagnosis of hypernephroma.

When Should You Request an Abdominal Echogram?

Ultrasound study of the abdomen may be useful in the following instances:
1. Evaluation of organomegaly.
2. To determine the fluid-filled or solid nature of a known abdominal mass.
3. To determine the presence, location, and relationships of abdominal masses (greater than 2 cm. in diameter).
4. Evaluation of the aorta. (May order aortic exam only.)
5. Radiation therapy or chemotherapy followup for change in size of tumor.
6. Examination of gallbladder for enlargement, response to fatty meal, presence of gallstones or tumor. Biliary radicles within the liver may also be seen. This is the only abdominal study that requires preparation. The patient should be NPO for 12 hours preceding the exam, and have a fat-free meal the evening before.
6a. Evaluation of jaundice; search for evidence of biliary tract obstruction.
7. Search for lymph node enlargement (greater than 2 cm. in diameter). Pelvic exam should also be requested.
8. Search for intra-abdominal or intraparenchymal abscess. Pelvic exam should also be requested.
9. Following trauma, to search for collections of blood around the spleen, kidney, liver, retroperitoneum, or within the abdominal cavity. Pelvic exam should also be requested.
10. Search for ascites. Pelvic exam should also be requested.
11. Search for retroperitoneal mass. Prone study should also be performed.

SUMMARY

1. When an ultrasound study of the abdomen is requested, most ultrasound departments will perform a supine study, beginning at the umbilicus and extending cephalad. A pelvic examination is not usually included unless specifically requested.

2. An abdominal study requires no special preparation, except that it cannot be performed for at least two days after an upper or lower GI series or an esophagogram (because of barium interference with transmission of the ultrasonic beam). Other types of x-ray contrast studies (intravenous pyelogram, oral cholecystogram, intravenous cholangiogram, angiogram) do not interfere with the ultrasound examination.

3. If disease is also suspected in the pelvis, pelvic exam should be requested. For an adequate pelvic exam the patient should ingest 16 to 24 ounces of fluid 30 to 45 minutes before the examination. This distends the bladder, displacing air-filled loops of bowel superiorly. The ultrasonographer then uses the bladder as an "ultrasonic window" through which to aim his transducer while searching for disease within the pelvis.

4. From a technical viewpoint, patients with many surgical dressings are difficult to scan because a satisfactory scan requires good contact between the skin and the transducer. Unsatisfactory scans also occur in patients with ileus or excessive intestinal gas from any cause. Patients in this latter group should be instructed to abstain from gas-producing foods and carbonated beverages for approximately 48 hours before the repeat scan is performed. Occasionally, simethicone is helpful in relieving gas.

CHAPTER 3

RENAL AND RETROPERITONEAL SCANNING

Up to this point, most of the abdominal echograms you have seen were obtained in the *supine* position. Although some kidney detail may be seen in this position, frequently all or part of a kidney may be obscured by intestinal gas. This is a simple problem to overcome, however, by scanning the patient in the *prone* position. As a matter of fact, you may think this sounds like a good idea for scanning *all* retroperitoneal structures. Think about it: the aorta and pancreas are retroperitoneal, but we usually scan them in the supine position. Why? What about the spleen? Bladder? Uterus?

There *is* a method to this madness. You have seen that both aorta and pancreas lie at least partially anterior to the vertebral bodies. The ultrasound beam is unable to penetrate bone, and therefore in the prone position any structures anterior to the spine are effectively "shadowed" from the beam. Similarly, pelvic structures such as bladder, prostate, and uterus cannot be seen in the prone position, owing to bony interference from the sacrum and iliac wings. The spleen and kidneys, however, lie lateral to the vertebral column, and therefore are commonly seen well in the prone position. The adrenal glands will be seen only if enlarged.

Figure 3–1*B* shows a *prone* transverse section obtained approximately 8 cm. above the iliac crest (IC+8), and Figure 3–1*A* is a line drawing of the section. The right side of the body is to the left of the picture. Again, you are looking down from the patient's head. The renal outlines and collecting system echoes are easily seen, as are the liver and slightly enlarged spleen. Note the lack of detail anterior to the vertebral body (acoustic shadowing). The stomach and intestines are not actually recognizable in this echogram, but are represented only by scattered echoes

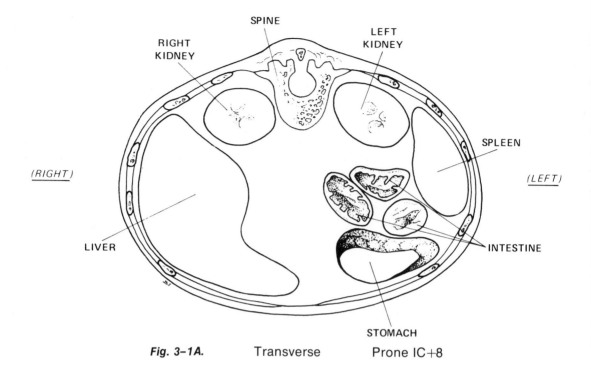

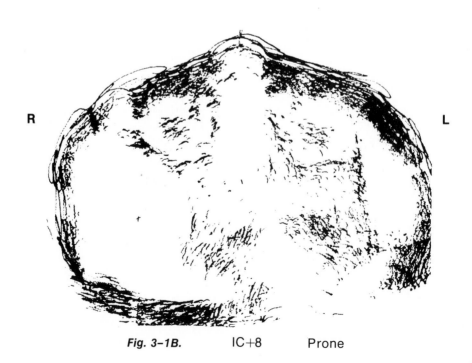

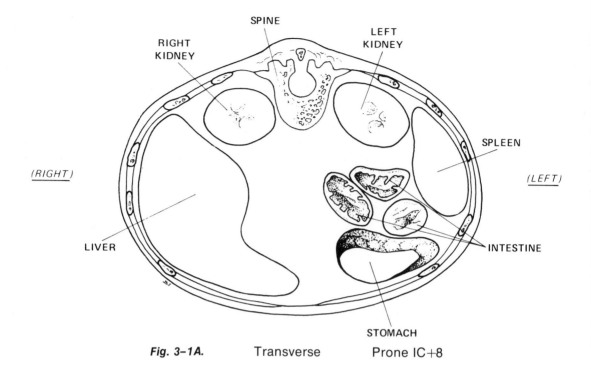

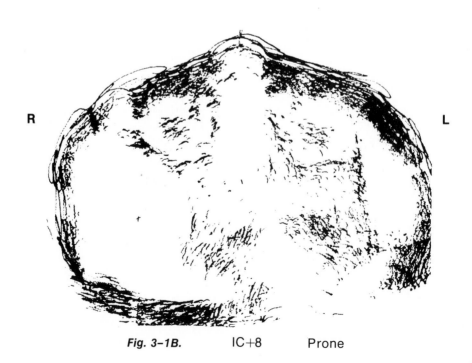

Fig. 3–1A.   Transverse   Prone IC+8

from the gas-filled loops of bowel. The tip of the left lobe of the liver could be delineated only by aiming the beam in from the right side through the liver substance. (Note the almost vertical orientation of the echoes outlining the liver tip. *The orientation of echoes is always perpendicular to the direction of the ultrasonic beam.*)

Fig. 3–1B.   IC+8   Prone

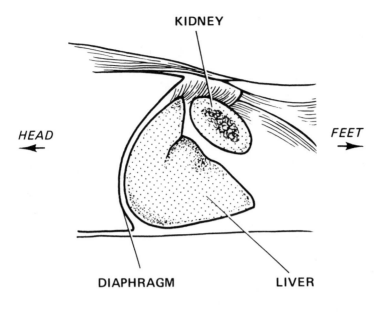

KIDNEY

HEAD ←

FEET →

DIAPHRAGM   LIVER

ANTERIOR

Fig. 3–2A.   Longitudinal   Prone R5

Figure 3–2B shows a prone longitudinal section of the right kidney, and Figure 3–2A is a line drawing of the section. You can tell it's the *right* kidney because you can see that it's nestled just beneath the liver. The echoes from the renal collecting system are grouped centrally, the normal appearance.

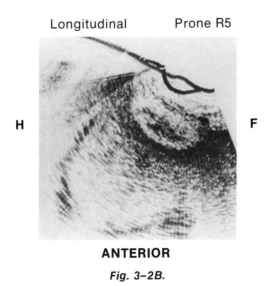

Longitudinal   Prone R5

H   F

ANTERIOR

Fig. 3–2B.

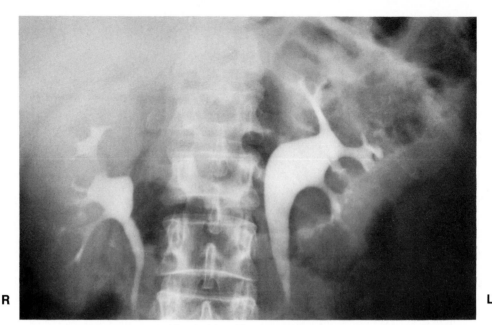

Fig. 3-3A. **Mr. Spraul's IVP**

Urban Spraul, the county assessor, who is 53 years old, comes to you for his annual physical. He is feeling well, and physical examination reveals no abnormalities. Urinalysis, however, shows microscopic hematuria.

THREE PATIENTS WITH HEMATURIA

Fig 3-4A. **Della's IVP**

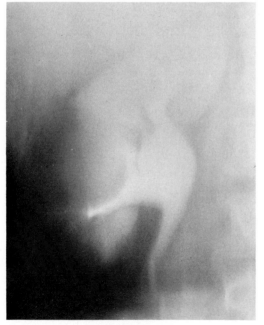

Courtesy of Dr. George Scher.

Right kidney

Della Terious is a 68-year-old Greek restaurant owner who has enjoyed generally good health. Within the past year, however, she has had two urinary tract infections. She once again comes to you, complaining of burning on urination. Physical examination is normal. Urinalysis reveals 18-20 WBC/HPF and 3-4 RBC/HPF.

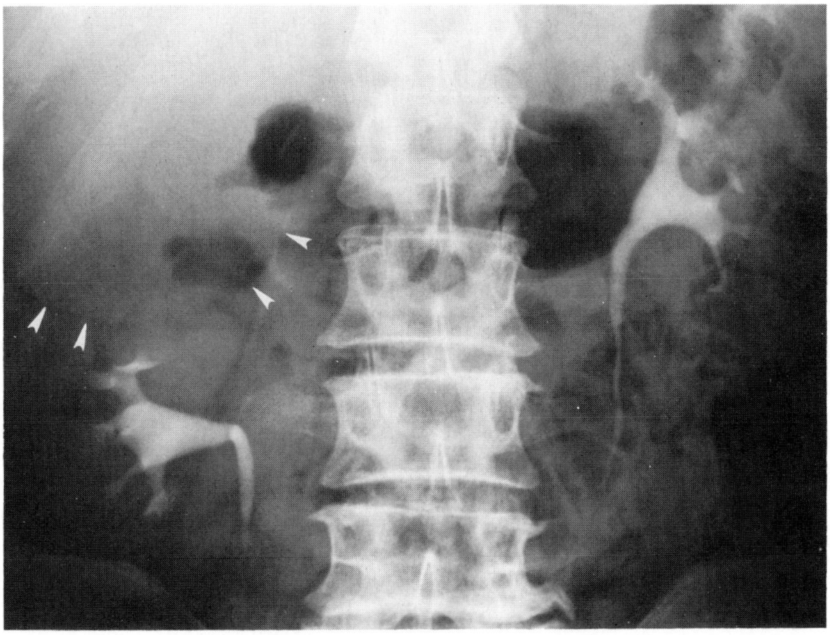

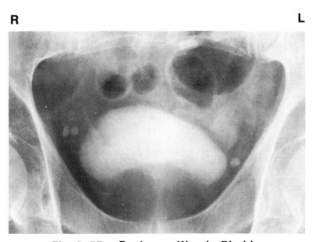

Fig. 3–5A. Professor Wood's IVP

Birnam Wood, 63, is a Shakespearean scholar. He complains of difficulty in maintaining his urinary stream. In addition, he awakens several times each night to void. Twice this week, he has noted a slight red tinge to his urine. Urinalysis confirms microscopic hematuria.

Fig. 3–5B. Professor Wood—Bladder

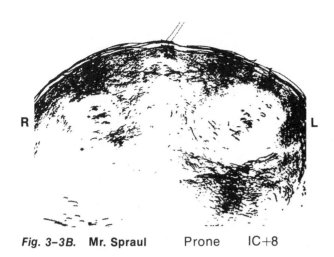

Fig. 3–3B. Mr. Spraul   Prone   IC+8

ANSWERS

Mr. Spraul's IVP (Fig. 3–3A) reveals a large, poorly outlined mass extending from the upper pole of his left kidney, spreading the infundibula apart. Faint calcification could be seen within the mass on the original film. This finding is very suggestive of a hypernephroma, although renal cysts rarely calcify. Now study the transverse echogram (Fig. 3–3B). Compare the size of the two kidneys, and notice the distribution of internal echoes. Remember: since the patient is *prone*, right and left are reversed from their positions on the supine scan.

POSTERIOR

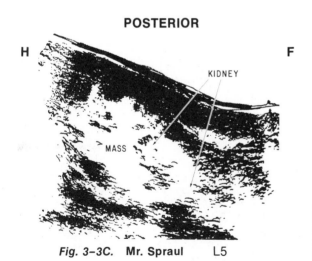

Fig. 3–3C. Mr. Spraul   L5

The longitudinal study (Fig. 3–3C) shows a large irregular mass extending cephalad and slightly posteriorly from the upper pole of the left kidney. On the transverse study, this mass is almost twice the volume of the right kidney at the same level. (Normal kidneys may show a *slight* disparity in size on a transverse section, since one kidney may be situated more inferiorly than the other, and the echogram therefore may not show comparable levels in each kidney.)

Note: On supine films of the abdomen, it is usually the *right* kidney that is situated more inferiorly. When the patient is in the prone position, however, the kidneys are at the same level in 50 per cent of patients.

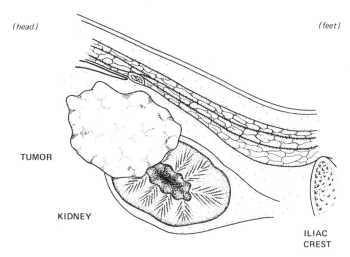

Fig. 3–3D. **Diagram. Left kidney**

The *internal* architecture of the two kidneys also differs markedly on the transverse echogram. The right kidney has a centrally located collection of strong echoes corresponding to the collecting system. On the left, the echoes are scattered throughout the mass, and vary from strong to weak. The longitudinal study shows organized collecting system echoes only in the lower pole. An arteriogram (Fig. 3–3E) confirmed the diagnosis of solid renal tumor. Note the characteristic tumor blush.

> TEACHING POINT: RENAL MASS WORK-UP. Localized calcifications within the kidney may occur in many conditions, including old healed tuberculosis, benign tumors, or renal cysts. However, *any renal mass containing calcium must be worked up for renal cell carcinoma, since such tumors often calcify, and resection may save the patient.*

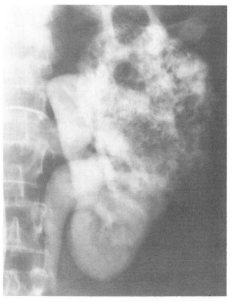

Fig. 3–3E. **Mr. Spraul's arteriogram (late phase)**

POSTERIOR

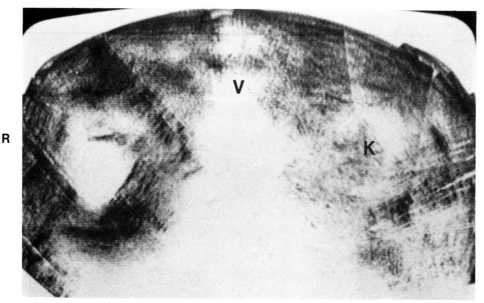

Fig. 3–4B. **Della**   Prone   IC+5

Della's IVP (Fig. 3–4A) shows a poorly defined mass extending from the anterolateral margin of her right lower pole. Even with nephrotomography, the right renal mass could not be optimally defined. It was thought to be cystic, however, and an echogram was requested to confirm this (Fig. 3–4B). On this transverse study through the lower poles of both kidneys, a sonolucent mass is seen anteriorly on the right. There is high through transmission beyond the mass. The left kidney (K) appears normal.

On the longitudinal study, (Fig. 3–4C) the mass displaces calyceal echoes posteriorly. This appearance (a sharply defined sonolucent mass with high through transmission) is characteristic of a renal cyst. The diagnosis was confirmed by cyst puncture. Della's hematuria, of course, was secondary to cystitis.

POSTERIOR

H

F

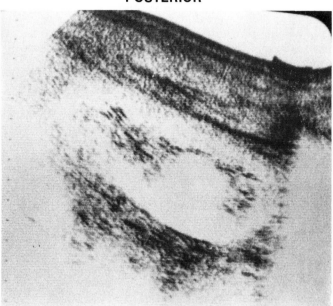

Fig. 3–4C. **Della's right kidney**   Prone

TEACHING POINT: RENAL MASS WORK-UP. In our hospitals, an echogram is the next step in the work-up for any renal mass seen at IVP, whether it is thought to be cystic or solid. If the echogram reveals a fluid-filled structure, cyst puncture is performed. (Very rarely, a renal tumor may arise within a cyst, or a necrotic tumor may appear to be fluid filled on ultrasound. In these cases, cyst puncture will usually reveal the presence of the tumor by abnormal cytology and/or a hemorrhagic aspirate. An angiogram is then performed.) If puncture is consistent with a diagnosis of renal cyst, no further work-up is necessary. On the other hand, if the echogram is equivocal or shows a solid renal mass, the work-up proceeds directly to angiography without cyst puncture. Since the vast majority of renal masses are cysts, and over 95 per cent of these are correctly diagnosed by ultrasound, many patients are saved the time, expense, and hazards (slight, but real) of angiography.

Professor Wood's IVP (Fig. 3–5*A*) shows a large right upper quadrant mass (arrows), displacing the kidney inferiorly. The renal outlines and collecting system, however, appear normal. Examination of the bladder (Fig. 3–5*B*) reveals prostatic enlargement, which confirms your findings on rectal examination. Episodes of gross hematuria may occasionally occur in patients with benign prostatic hypertrophy.

L R

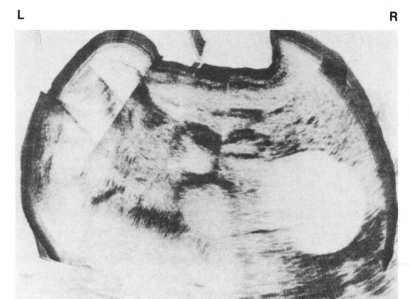

Fig. 3–5C. **Professor Wood**

Supine U+14

H F

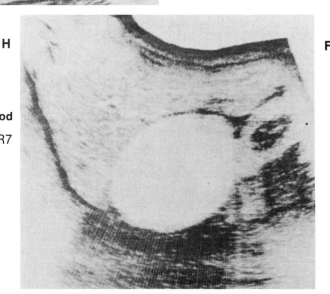

Fig. 3–5D. **Professor Wood**

Supine R7

Now study *Professor Wood's* transverse (Fig. 3–5C) and longitudinal (Fig. 3–5D) echograms. The mass is clearly superior to the upper pole of the right kidney, and appears cystic rather than solid. Because of its location, an adrenal cyst is the most likely possibility; however, a hepatic cyst cannot be completely excluded on these studies. Cyst puncture revealed clear fluid with no abnormal cells. The cyst was drained, but repeat echogram performed three weeks after puncture (Fig. 3–5E) showed some reaccumulation of fluid.

Three weeks later

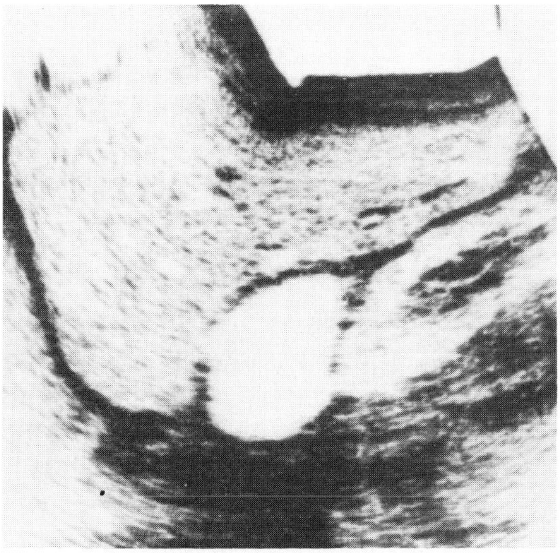

Fig. 3–5E. **Professor Wood**   R7

Ben Dover is a 44-year-old high school athletic director who has been under treatment for lymphoma. He comes to the Ultrasound Department every six months for a routine search for enlarged abdominal nodes. This time, he also complains of some right-sided back pain. His next clinic appointment is in four weeks.

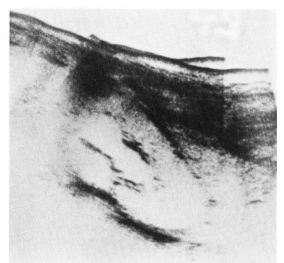

H   F

Fig. 3–6A. **Ben Longitudinal right kidney** Prone

THREE PATIENTS WITH BACK PAIN

Supine   U+10

Gloria Mundy, 52, ambulance service owner (motto: Sick Transit? Gloria Mundy!), had surgery for bronchogenic carcinoma one year ago. Recently she has been feeling tired and has had some vague pain in the upper lumbar region. She is thin, and appears chronically ill. Lumbar spine films are normal.

L   *Fig. 3–7A.* **Mrs. Mundy**   R

L   R

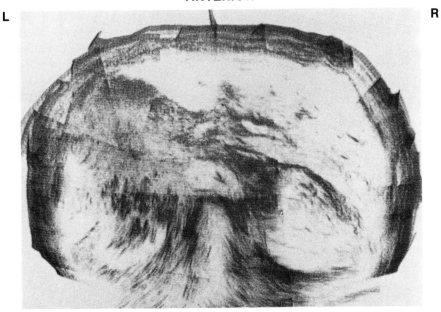

Fig. 3–8A. **Mr. Liebknecht**   Supine U+12

Gerhard Liebknecht, the violin maker, has lost 10 pounds in the last three months. His wife is worried. At age 62, he still attacks her dumplings and wurst with gusto, but he's always been plump and she likes him that way. In addition, lately he's been kept awake at night by severe right-sided back pain. Physical exam shows a slightly obese, but otherwise perfectly normal man. Since it's Friday afternoon, the only test you can get right away is an echogram. This study was done supine.

ANSWERS

Fig. 3–6B. **Ben**

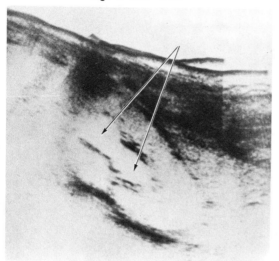

H   **Prone right kidney**   F

Ben had a fair amount of intestinal gas, which precluded optimal visualization of enlarged nodes on the supine study. The technologist noted an abnormal appearance of his right kidney and turned him to the *prone* position for further evaluation (Fig. 3–6B). The calyceal pattern is unusual. This appearance is characteristic of a distended renal pelvis. The dark echoes arise from the outer surface of the renal pelvis, and the central, clear area (arrows) represents the fluid within.

IVP (Fig. 3–6C) confirmed the ultrasonic diagnosis of right renal obstruction, presumably due to enlarged pelvic nodes. Later echograms (with less gaseous interference) revealed enlarged nodes in the right side of the pelvis.

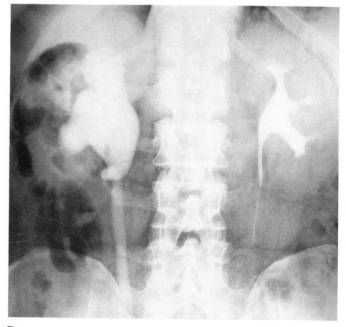

R   *Fig. 3–6C.* **Ben's IVP**   L

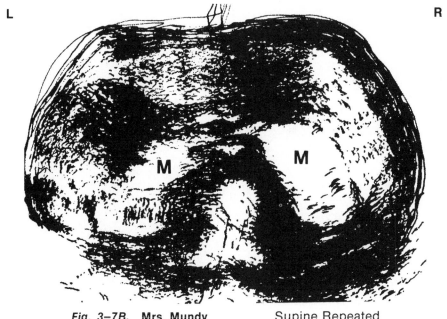

L   R

Fig. 3–7B. **Mrs. Mundy**   Supine Repeated

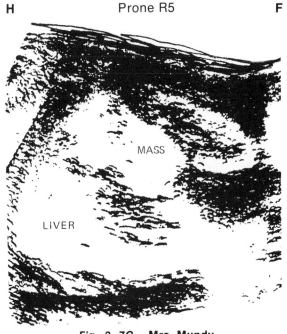

H   Prone R5   F

Fig. 3–7C. **Mrs. Mundy**

Two relatively sonolucent masses (M) can be seen (one anterior to each kidney) on *Mrs. Mundy's* supine echogram (Fig. 3–7B). The masses have few internal echoes; however, there is no evidence of high through transmission. These findings suggest relatively homogeneous solid lesions. Prone longitudinal view (Fig. 3–7C) reveals that the mass on the right extends anterosuperior to the kidney. A similar appearance was seen on the left (not shown). The lesions proved to be adrenal metastases, a not uncommon sequel of bronchogenic carcinoma.

L   R

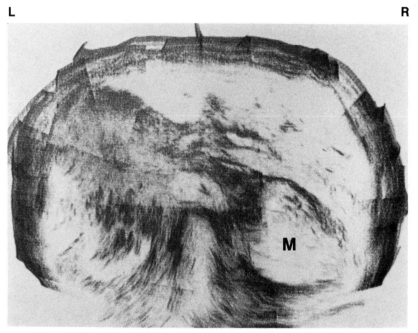

Fig. 3–8B. **Mr. Liebknecht**   Transverse Repeated

Mr. Liebknecht's echogram (Fig. 3–8B) shows an unusual renal pattern. His right upper pole (M) is enlarged (compare with the left), and contains occasional fine internal echoes. On the supine longitudinal projection (Fig. 3–8C), a large mass (M) can be seen extending superiorly from the right kidney.

H   F

Fig. 3–8C. **Mr. Liebknecht**

Supine R6

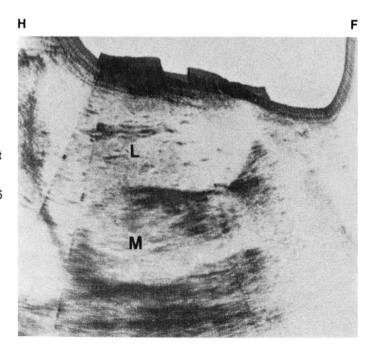

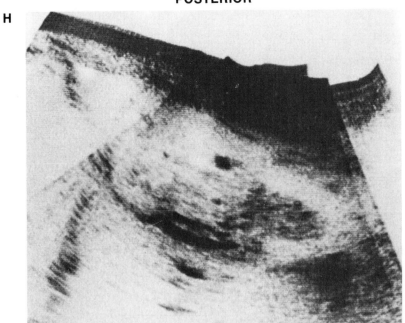

Fig. 3–8D. **Mr. Liebknecht**   Prone   R6

ANSWERS — *Continued*

The mass is delineated even better on the *prone* view (Figs. 3–8D and 3–8E). At surgery, the entire right upper pole was found to be replaced by a hypernephroma.

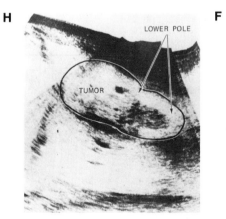

Fig. 3–8E. **Mr. Liebknecht's renal tumor**

TWO CHILDREN WHO PRESENT WITH AN ABDOMINAL MASS

L   ANTERIOR   R

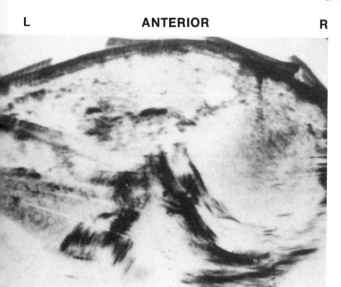

Fig. 3–9A. **Brockley**   Supine Transverse

Brockley Parsnip, age 15 months, is the scion of a West Coast health food chain. While bathing Brockley one day, his mother noticed a hard mass on the right side of his abdomen. Your physical examination confirms the mass, which seems inseparable from the liver and extends to the level of the umbilicus. *Note:* All of Brockley's echograms were performed with the patient in the supine position.

H   ANTERIOR   F

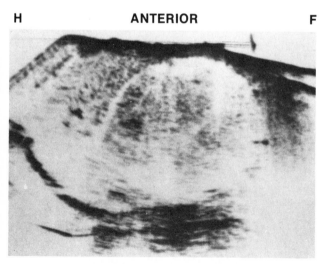

Fig. 3–9B. **Brockley**   Longitudinal Supine

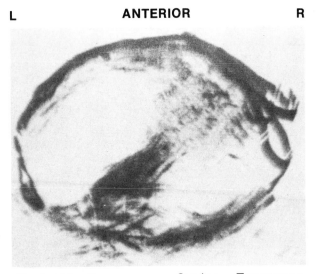

Fig. 3–10A. **Duncan**   Supine   Transverse

Duncan Fife, 10 days old, is brought to the Emergency Room one evening by his worried parents. While tickling the baby, his father felt a mass in the left abdomen. Your physical examination reveals *bilateral* poorly defined, doughy masses. *Duncan's* echograms were also performed in the supine position.

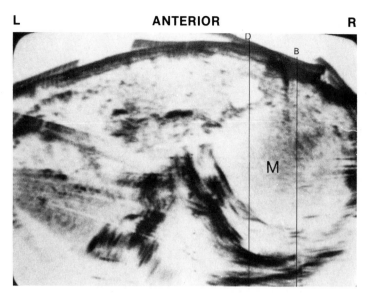

Fig. 3–9C. **Brockley**   Transverse   Repeated

ANSWERS

Transverse and longitudinal echograms of young *Brockley's* abdomen show a large, round mass (M) with multiple internal echoes. The mass extends to the level of the umbilicus (indicated by the electronic marker on the longitudinal study), and is clearly separable from the liver. What is the rounded lucency located anteriorly on the transverse scan? When a longitudinal section (Fig. 3–9D) was obtained through the area of this lucency, it was seen to be the gallbladder, somewhat displaced by the large mass. (The planes of both longitudinal sections are indicated by lines B and D.)

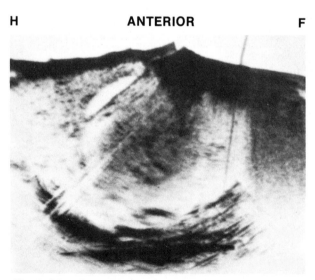

Fig. 3–9D. **Brockley**   Longitudinal (plane D)

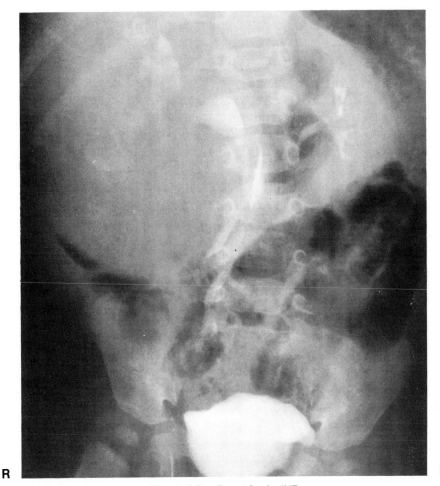

R   L

Fig. 3–9E. **Brockley's IVP**

Since the right kidney could not be identified on the echogram, an intravenous pyelogram (Fig. 3–9E) was obtained. This shows a huge mass involving the entire right abdomen, displacing bowel gas inferiorly and to the left. The collecting system of the right kidney is distorted, and the ureter is also displaced medially.

Brockley did well after the surgeons removed a large Wilms' tumor. He was lucky on two counts: 1) generally, the chances of survival with a Wilms' tumor are much worse when the tumor occurs in a child older than two years; and 2) five to 10 per cent of Wilms' tumors are bilateral. Brockley's wasn't. Yet.

L   **ANTERIOR**   R

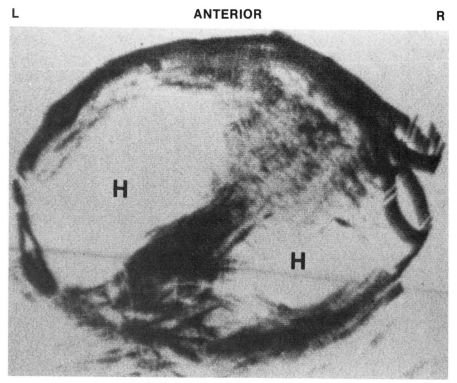

Fig. 3–10B. **Duncan**   Transverse Repeated

The transverse echogram of *Duncan's* abdomen was difficult to perform because of the baby's squirming. That's why the vertebral column and great vessels are not clearly delineated. No amount of motion, however, could conceal the large, *bilateral*, sonolucent masses (H) filling both sides of the abdominal cavity. As the kidneys could not be outlined, massive hydronephrosis was suspected.

Duncan's intravenous pyelogram (Fig. 3–10C) shows dilatation of the renal collecting systems bilaterally. The right renal pelvis and calyces are densely outlined by contrast material. On the left, you can also see a huge saclike collection of contrast material (arrows), less dense than on the right side. This represents a mixture of urine and contrast material in the obstructed left collecting system. This appearance suggests that the obstruction on the left is even greater than that on the right, allowing a large amount of unopacified urine to be retained, mixing with the contrast. This produces a more distended, but less opacified renal collecting system on the left.

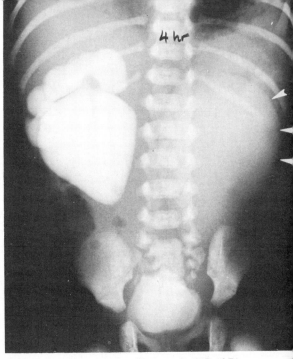

R   *Fig. 3–10C.* **Duncan's IVP (AP)**

The lateral view from the intravenous pyelogram (Fig. 3–10D) also shows dense contrast in the right collecting system. The less dense (but larger) mass of the left collecting system extends anteriorly (arrows). This also confirms the echographic appearance, which showed the mass on the left to be nearly twice as large as that on the right. The ureters were never seen well, although the bladder did fill with contrast.

Duncan had bilateral ureteropelvic junction obstruction, which was relieved by surgery. Ureteropelvic junction obstruction and multicystic kidney are probably the two most common causes of unilateral flank mass in a neonate. Duncan was unfortunate in having bilateral disease.

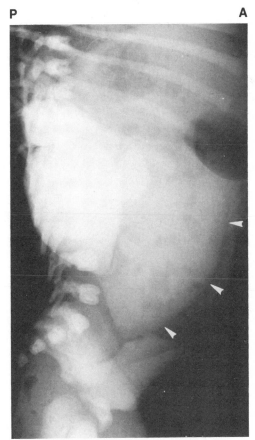

Fig. 3–10D. **Duncan's IVP (Lateral)**

THE CASE OF THE DISAPPEARING CYST

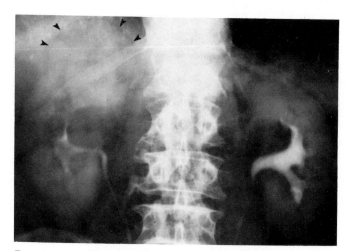

R   *Fig. 3–11A.* **Miss Swann's IVP**   **L**

Odette Swann, 52, ballet teacher, had an intravenous pyelogram (Fig. 3–11A) as part of her work-up for recurrent urinary tract infections. A right upper pole mass (arrows) was identified, and echography recommended.

H   **POSTERIOR**   **F**

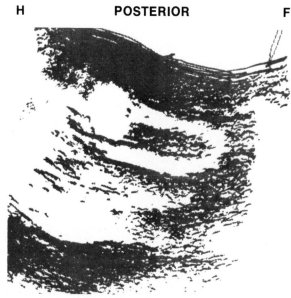

Fig. 3–11B. **Miss Swann's right kidney**

Longitudinal echogram (Fig. 3–11B) revealed a well-demarcated, sonolucent mass involving the posterior aspect of the right upper pole. At high gain (not shown), there was no evidence of internal echoes. These findings are characteristic of a fluid-filled lesion, such as a renal cyst. In order to confirm this diagnosis, however, cyst puncture was scheduled.

On the day of the cyst puncture, the cyst was again localized with ultrasound, and its position marked on the patient's skin. The patient then received an intravenous injection of IVP contrast material, and cyst puncture was performed under fluoroscopic control. (Cyst puncture may also be performed under ultrasound control, using a special biopsy transducer with a central hole for passage of the needle.)

H   **PRONE**   **F**

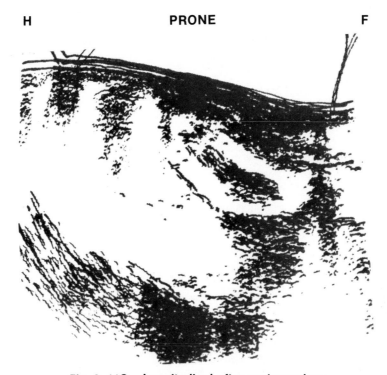

Fig. 3–11C. **Longitudinal after cyst puncture**

Much to everyone's surprise, no fluid could be aspirated despite multiple attempts. Repeat echogram (Fig. 3–11C) was even more disconcerting. There was no trace of the mass, only a few echoes where it used to be.

DISAPPEARING CYST – Continued

Fig. 3–11D. **Miss Swann's right kidney**

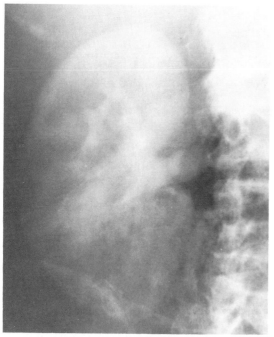

Arteriogram (Nephrogram phase)

The patient then underwent an angiogram (Fig. 3–11D), which also showed no trace of the previously noted right upper pole mass. Where had it gone? It was postulated that during the initial attempt at puncture, the cyst was entered by the needle, but that the tip of the needle had gone beyond the fluid-filled area. When the needle was withdrawn, fluid leaked out, accounting for the later unsuccessful attempts.

When *Miss Swann* returned for her check-up several weeks later, we were eager to repeat her ultrasound exam (Fig. 3–11E). Of course, the cyst had reaccumulated fluid and looked just as it had at the beginning. Miss Swann declined another diagnostic tap and returned to her pliés. Most of the time, cyst puncture is a rapid and easy procedure. Not always.

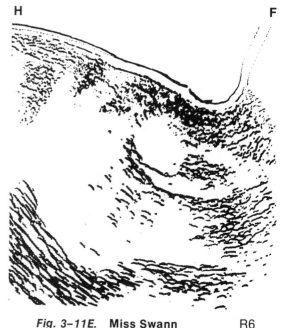

Fig. 3–11E. **Miss Swann** R6

A PATIENT WITH HYPERTENSION

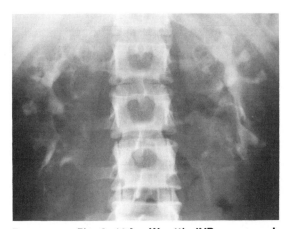

R**Fig. 3–12A.** **Wyatt's IVP** L

Courtesy of Dr. Lee Talner

Wyatt Ahl is depressed at 23. After losing his job, he decided to join the Army. But even the Army turned him down. They did, however, advise him to seek treatment for his hypertension. Wyatt's blood pressure is 170/100. He tells you that his mother (now deceased) also had high blood pressure.

Wyatt's IVP (Fig. 3–12A) shows massive enlargement of both kidneys, with marked distortion of the collecting systems due to pressure from adjacent cysts.

R   L

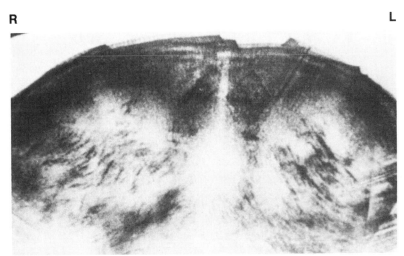

Fig. 3–12B.

Prone   IC+6

Transverse (Fig. 3–12B) and longitudinal (Fig. 3–12C) echograms confirm the diagnosis of polycystic kidneys. Note the large size of the kidneys and the multiple sonolucent masses within. Echograms of Wyatt's liver (not shown) also showed occasional cysts. Adult polycystic kidney disease always involves both kidneys, although the involvement may not be symmetrical. Liver cysts occur in approximately one third of patients, and cysts in other organs (pancreas, lungs) may also occur.

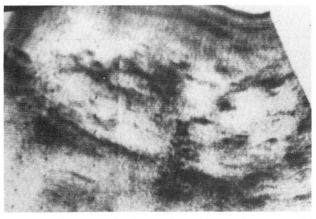

H   **Fig. 3–12C.** **Left kidney (close-up)** F

CHECKLIST FOR ABDOMINAL AND RETROPERITONEAL ECHOGRAPHY

	INDICATION	STUDY	PREPARATION	INTERFERENCE
1.	Organomegaly	Abdomen	None	Overlying dressings, intestinal gas, barium
2.	Known abdominal mass (determine fluid or solid nature, relationship to other organs)	Abdomen	None	Overlying dressings, intestinal gas, barium
3.	Suspected abdominal mass (especially pancreas) (determine presence, location, fluid or solid)	Abdomen	None	Overlying dressings, intestinal gas, barium
4.	Suspected aortic aneurysm	Aorta	None	Overlying dressings, intestinal gas, barium
5.	Radiation or chemotherapy follow-up	Depends on area of interest	2–3 glasses (8 oz.) of fluid 45 minutes before exam to fill bladder (if searching for pelvic nodes)	Overlying dressings, intestinal gas, barium
6.	Cholelithiasis	Gallbladder	Fat-free meal evening before exam. NPO 12 hours preceding exam	Overlying dressings, intestinal gas, barium
6a.	Jaundice (precluding satisfactory oral cholecystogram)	Abdomen Gallbladder	Fat-free meal evening before exam. NPO 12 hours preceding exam	Overlying dressings, intestinal gas, barium
7.	Suspected lymph node enlargement (>2 cm.)	Abdomen Pelvis	2–3 glasses (8 oz.) of fluid 45 minutes before exam	Overlying dressings, intestinal gas, barium
8.	Search for intra-abdominal or intraparenchymal abscess	Abdomen (including views of diaphragmatic motion) Pelvis	2–3 glasses (8 oz.) of fluid 45 minutes before exam	Overlying dressings, intestinal gas, barium
8a.	Suspected perinephric abscess	Kidneys (prone)	None	Overlying dressings, intestinal gas, barium
9.	Abdominal trauma (suspect hematoma: retroperitoneal, renal, hepatic, splenic; or free blood in abdominal cavity)	Abdomen Pelvis Retroperitoneum (prone)	None	Overlying dressings, intestinal gas, barium
10.	Ascites	Abdomen Pelvis	None	Overlying dressings, intestinal gas, barium
11.	Suspected retroperitoneal mass	Abdomen Pelvis Retroperitoneum (prone) (depends on suspected area)	2–3 glasses (8 oz.) of fluid 45 minutes before exam (if searching for pelvic involvement)	Overlying dressings, intestinal gas, barium
12.	Renal mass evaluation	Kidneys (prone)	IVP	Overlying dressings, intestinal gas, barium

CHAPTER 4

OBSTETRIC AND GYNECOLOGIC SCANNING

Once the basic principles of B-scanning are understood, it is easy to see how important this technique can be in the evaluation of obstetric and gynecologic problems. This is particularly true in view of the physician's natural hesitancy about irradiating a developing fetus or the gonads of a woman still in her reproductive years. Although studies to date have proven no deleterious effects from ultrasound used at the intensity levels commonly employed for diagnostic purposes, it is the physician's responsibility to use the technique judiciously (i.e., only if there is a medical indication for its use). It should *not* be used, as has happened occasionally, merely as a confirmation of the fetal presence, to please the proud parents.

A full bladder is necessary for satisfactory pelvic scanning. The bladder displaces the bowel superiorly and thus provides an "ultrasonic window" through which to aim the beam for better visualization of pelvic organs. The pregnant uterus (or any large pelvic mass) may actually be elevated somewhat superiorly by the full bladder, allowing better visualization of its contours.

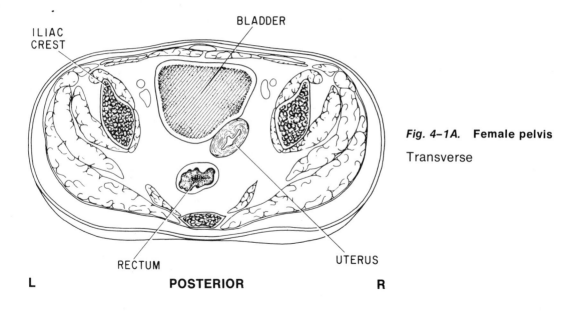

BLADDER

Fig. 4–1A.   Female pelvis

Transverse

RECTUM

UTERUS

L   **POSTERIOR**   R

Figure 4–1B shows a transverse echogram obtained at a level approximately 4 cm. superior to the symphysis pubis (S+4) in a normal nonpregnant female. Figure 4–1A is a line drawing of the section. The uterus is displaced slightly to the right. This small amount of lateral displacement of the uterine fundus is a normal variant. The adnexa are not seen in this patient. The normal adnexa usually measure less than 2 cm. in diameter, which is the lower limit of resolution of the ultrasound beam. In most cases, therefore, the adnexa can be seen by ultrasound only if they are enlarged.

Transverse   S+4

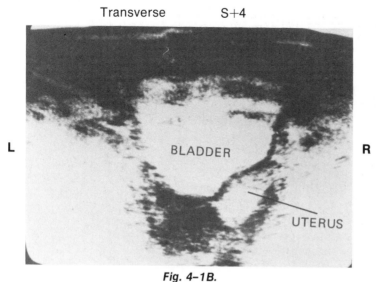

L   BLADDER   R

UTERUS

Fig. 4–1B.

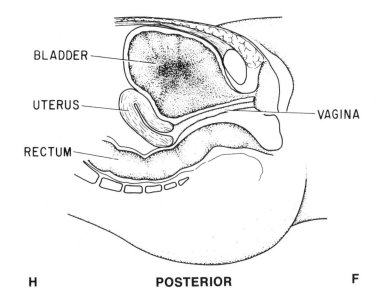

Fig. 4–2A. **Female pelvis**

Longitudinal

BLADDER

UTERUS

RECTUM

VAGINA

H   **POSTERIOR**   **F**

Figure 4–2B is a longitudinal study of the same patient, and Figure 4–2A is the corresponding line drawing. Note the linear horizontal echo of the cervical canal.

> *Hint:* On gray scale studies, you can ignore the artefactual echoes present anteriorly in fluid-filled structures (e.g., bladder) which lie just below the skin surface.

H   Longitudinal   F

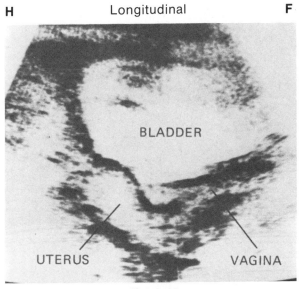

BLADDER

UTERUS

VAGINA

Fig. 4–2B.

THE MISSING STRINGS

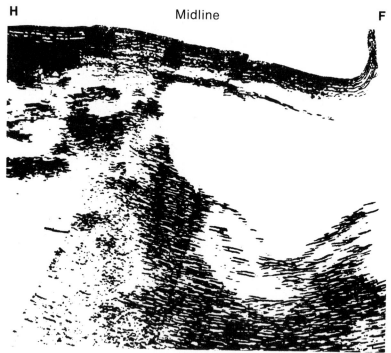

H Midline F

Fig. 4–3A. **Sherry**

Toastmistress **Sherry Wine,** 38, has worn her IUD successfully for three years. Recently she noticed that she could no longer feel the string.

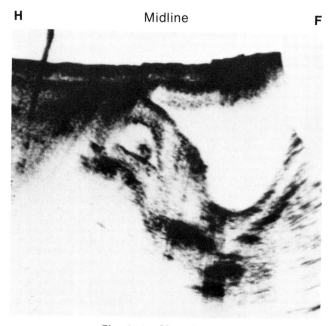

H Midline F

Fig. 4–4. **Miss Fiasco**

Winifred Fiasco, 32, coloratura, has a similar problem, with one additional complication: in addition to missing her string, she confides to you that she has also missed her period, but only once. She is due to menstruate this week, but is a little late....

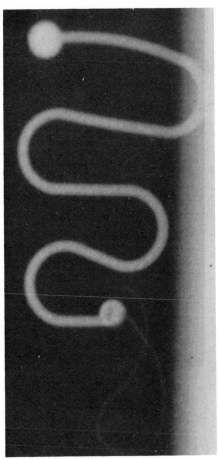

Fig. 4–3B. **Sherry's IUD**

ANSWERS

Sherry was relieved to learn that her IUD (Fig. 4–3B) was in satisfactory position within the uterine cavity. On the echogram (Fig. 4–3A) it appears as multiple strong echoes reflected from the parallel turns of the device.

Miss Fiasco's echogram (Fig. 4–4), however, tells a different story. Her uterus is enlarged, and there is a tear-drop-shaped, sonolucent sac in the fundus. This represents the gestational sac, and the small echoes within it are from the developing fetus. Note the good visualization of the vaginal canal. Where was the IUD? It was still in the uterus (but not seen in this particular section), and was delivered along with the baby about 32 weeks following this ultrasound examination.

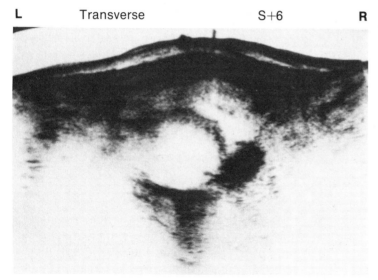

Fig. 4–5A. **Mrs. Jenn**

Esther Jenn, who is now 30, had her uterus removed during the course of her sixth C-section five years ago. Now, during her routine checkup, you feel a nontender pelvic mass, just to the left of the midline.

FOUR PATIENTS WITH PELVIC MASSES

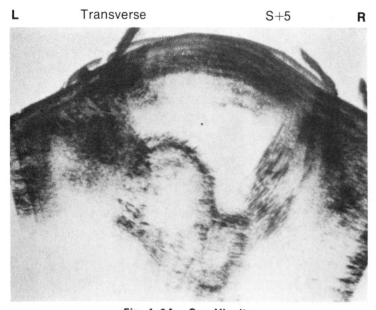

Fig. 4–6A. **Sra. Vincitor**

Ritorna Vincitor, 43, aging femme fatale currently filming in the U. S., has been bothered by irregular periods for the last eight months. As film crew physician, you examine her and note a large, firm mass inseparable from the uterus. The mass is nontender and extends slightly to the left. Well, you *didn't* transport a B-scanner into the Mojave Desert with you, but fortunately civilization lies only 40 minutes away by air.

At age 19, typist **Bunny Love** supports a $100 a day drug habit. She is a generous young woman, however, and right now she regrets it. She comes to the Free Clinic in tears, with marked pelvic tenderness and recent exacerbation of her vaginal discharge. Because of her pain, you cannot perform an adequate pelvic examination, but you *think* you feel a mass in the cul-de-sac.

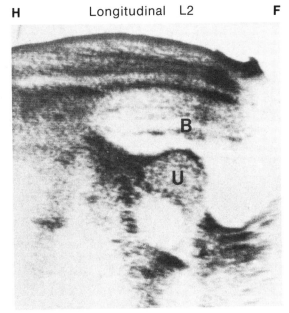

Fig. 4–7A. Bunny

Superior Court Judge **Fay Semple**, 27, is approximately three months pregnant. Her previous pregnancy ended in a miscarriage, and now she again has reason to worry. Last evening she noticed some spotting. Your physical examination shows her uterus to be about the same size it was two weeks ago. Or maybe it's a little smaller.

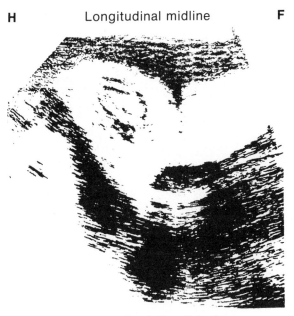

Fig. 4–8A. Judge Semple

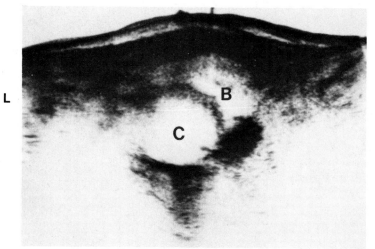

L

R

Transverse Repeated
S+6

Fig. 4–5B. **Mrs. Jenn**

ANSWERS

Esther's transverse echogram (Fig. 4–5B) shows a round, sonolucent mass (C) with a sharp distal border and good through transmission, lying posterior to the bladder and to the left. These findings are characteristics of a fluid-filled mass, and are confirmed on the longitudinal study (Fig. 4–5C). The uterus, of course, is surgically absent. The diagnosis of left ovarian cyst was confirmed at surgery.

H   **ANTERIOR**   F

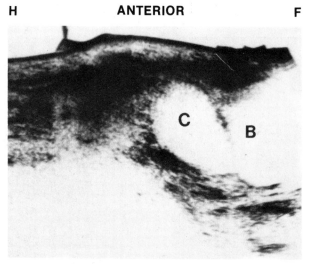

Longitudinal   L3

Fig. 4–5C. **Mrs. Jenn**

ANTERIOR

Transverse Repeated

L

R

L

Fig. 4–6B. Sra. Vincitor   S+5

ANSWERS — *Continued*

The transverse echogram (Fig. 4–6B) on *Sra. Vincitor* showed, as expected, a large solid mass (L) inseparable from the uterus and indenting the posterior portion of the bladder on the left. There are fine echoes within the mass, and the posterior border is poorly defined. There is little through transmission, in contrast with the appearance expected with a fluid-filled mass. (Compare Figure 4–5B, *Mrs. Jenn.*) This appearance is entirely compatible with a diagnosis of leiomyomata. Similar findings are seen on the longitudinal study (Fig. 4–6C).

H   **ANTERIOR**   F

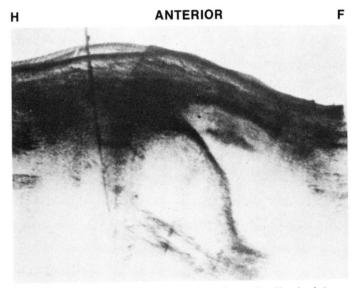

Fig. 4–6C. Sra. Vincitor   Longitudinal L1

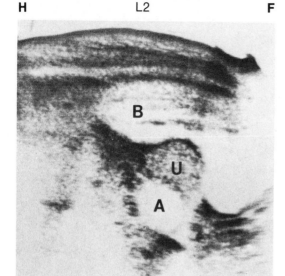

H   L2   F

Fig. 4–7B. **Bunny**

Longitudinal repeated

ANSWERS – *Continued*

Bunny's longitudinal echogram (Fig. 4–7B) reveals a fluid-filled mass (A) lying posterior to the uterus (U), displacing it anteriorly. (Again, see how clear the difference is between the solid uterus and the fluid-filled mass. This difference would be far less obvious using bistable technique.) Additional longitudinal scans and a transverse scan (Fig. 4–7C) showed there were actually *two* fluid-filled structures, each lying posterolaterally to the uterus. If you're thinking about bilateral tubo-ovarian abscesses, you're *right*.

ANTERIOR

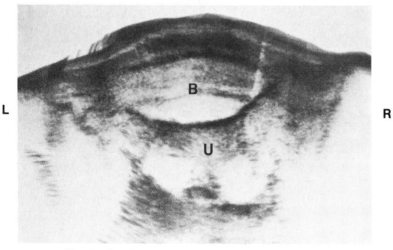

L   R

Fig. 4–7C. **Bunny**   Transverse   S+5

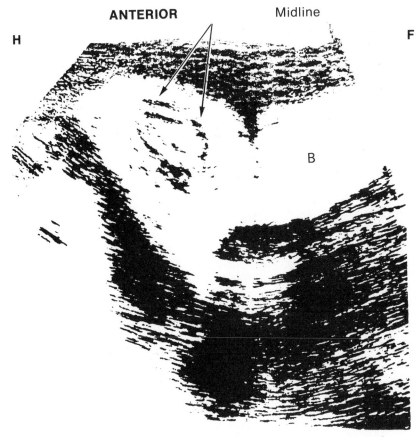

ANTERIOR   Midline

H   F

B

Fig. 4–8B. **Judge Semple**   Longitudinal repeated

Examination of *Judge Semple's* echogram (Fig. 4–8B) shows an enlarged uterus containing an irregular incomplete ring of echoes (arrows) in the fundus. This represents the disintegrating gestational sac usually recognizable with impending abortion. The normal gestational sac is a slightly oval, well-defined complete ring of echoes. When a gestational sac becomes irregular in shape, fragmented, or in low position in the uterus, fetal demise should be suspected. Compare this picture with Figure 4–4 (Winifred Fiasco, p. 100). Note how the gray scale picture shows many fine echoes from the uterine wall (thickened by proliferation of decidual cells) surrounding the sac. These fine echoes are below the threshold of resolution on the bistable picture.

The Placenta

The echographer is frequently called upon to determine the position of the placenta, either in patients with suspected placenta previa, or in patients in whom amniocentesis is to be performed. Placental localization by echographic techniques is almost 100 per cent accurate, limited only by the skill of the persons performing and interpreting the study. It is the position of the fetus itself that gives the first clue to the position of the placenta. If the fetus is lying against the anterior wall of the uterus, for instance, one should be prepared to find a posterior placenta.

The placenta itself usually shows a sharply defined fetal border, representing the chorionic plate. Its internal structure produces a stippled pattern of echoes, particularly evident on gray scale pictures. Usually, in any one section, only portions of the fetus may be seen. Occasionally, as in the accompanying illustration (Fig. 4–9), the beam will traverse the entire fetus in longitudinal section, and then both head and trunk may be outlined in the same picture.

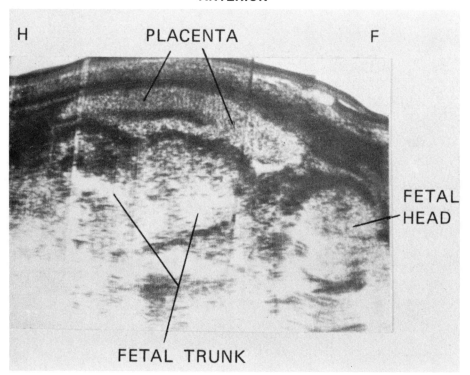

Fig. 4–9. **Placenta**

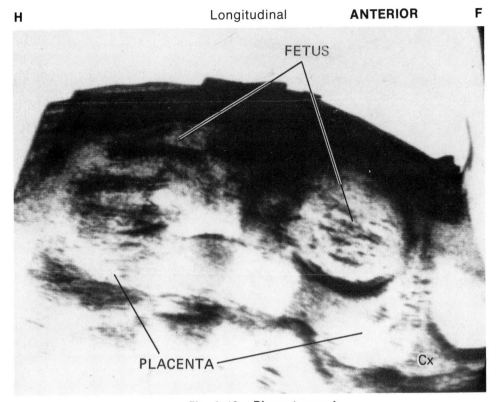

Fig. 4-10. **Placenta previa**

Commonly, a posteriorly placed placenta is less well defined than an anterior one, owing to "shadowing" of the internal structure by the fetal body. That is, so much of the sound energy is taken up in traversing the body of the fetus that there is little sound energy left to delineate the internal architecture of the posterior placenta (Fig. 4-10). In this patient the fetal head is displaced out of the pelvis by a posterior placenta previa. Note the position of the cervix.

TOTAL CENTRAL PLACENTA PREVIA

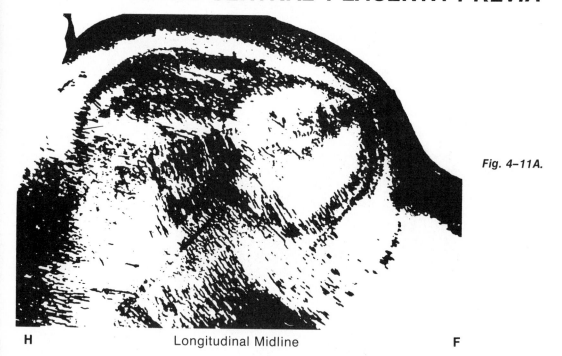

Fig. 4–11A.

H   Longitudinal Midline   F

In patients with total central placenta previa, the entire fetus may be displaced superiorly into the uterine fundus (Fig. 4–11A and B). In this picture, note the thin uterine wall separating the back of the fetus from the maternal abdominal wall. Compare this with the thick band of placental tissue (containing fine internal echoes) that separates the fetal head from the maternal bladder.

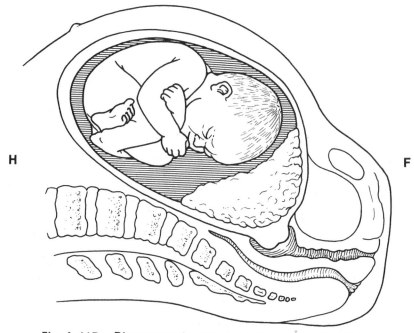

H   F

Fig. 4–11B. **Diagrammatic representation of Fig. 4–11A**

BIPARIETAL DIAMETER

The fetal skull is visible in 95 per cent of cases by the thirteenth or fourteenth week of gestation. Fetal age can be accurately determined echographically by measurement of the greatest biparietal diameter. This measurement is usually performed in transverse scans, with the transducer angle adjusted so that the baby's falx shows as a single line extending anteroposteriorly across the midline of the skull (Fig. 4–12). Note the finely stippled placenta lying anteriorly.

L   Transverse   R

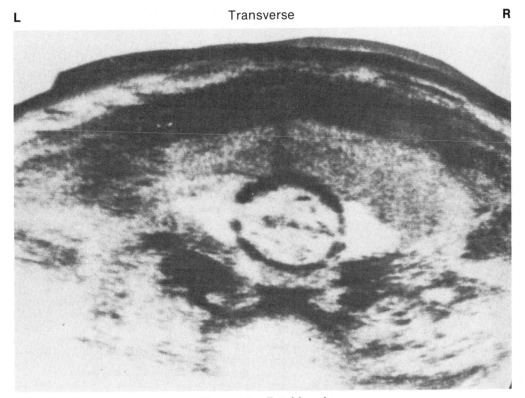

Fig. 4–12. **Fetal head**

The falx echo is ordinarily seen well only when the fetal biparietal diameter is traversed. Gestational age can be determined more accurately by measuring the biparietal diameter than by other methods (history, palpation, x-rays). When accurate determination of fetal maturity is of great importance in a patient near term, this technique may also be used in conjunction with the lecithin-sphingomyelin ratio of the amniotic fluid. (An appropriate site for amniotic fluid withdrawal is localized by ultrasound). An L/S ratio greater than 2:1 indicates maturity of the fetal lungs.

OVERSIZE PROBLEMS

ANTERIOR

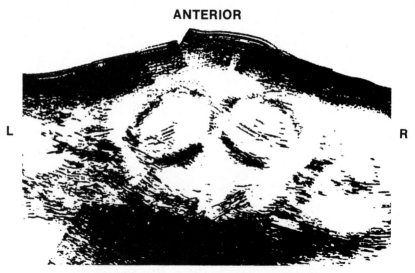

L   R

Fig. 4–13A. **Gemini Farout— 6 Months**

The 25-year-old astrologer **Gemini Farout** conceived when the signs were right. Now she's in her sixth month of pregnancy, but any casual observer would have guessed it was her tenth.

H   Longitudinal   F

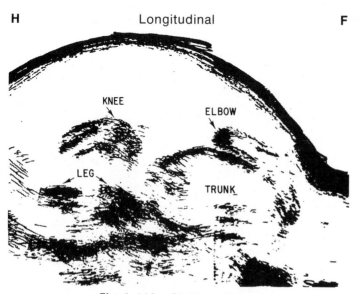

KNEE

ELBOW

LEG

TRUNK

Fig. 4–14A. **Siobhan O'Hara**

(Modified from Leopold and Asher, Radiologic Clinics of North America, Vol. XI, No. 1, April 1974.)

Playwright **Siobhan O'Hara** lost her first child 20 years ago, when she was 23, owing to what she mysteriously tells you is "the family curse." She has had three perfectly normal children since, and is now happily pregnant again. She *is* big for her dates, and is praying for twins.

ANTERIOR

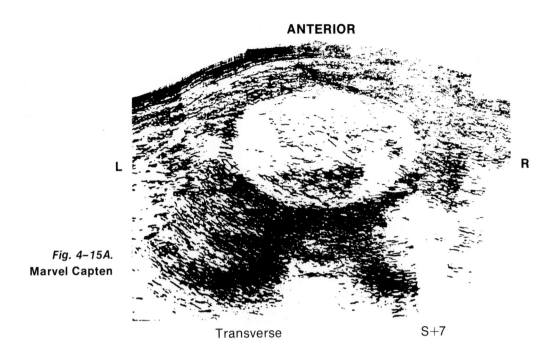

L   R

Fig. 4–15A.
Marvel Capten

Transverse   S+7

Marvel Capten, 22, has never been pregnant before. She and her husband are both graduate students, and because of financial difficulties she did not seek prenatal care. She's in her fifth month of pregnancy and is concerned because her friends say she should "feel life" by now. On examination her uterus is approximately six months' size, but you cannot hear fetal heart tones.

Ida Clare, the fashion expert for "Unwrinkled Charm" (a women's wear daily), is 32 and has been diabetic for 16 years. Her previous baby weighed 13 pounds at birth. Ida has a strong tendency to deny her health problems, and now comes to you in her ninth month of pregnancy. She has not felt fetal movement for three days and is worried.

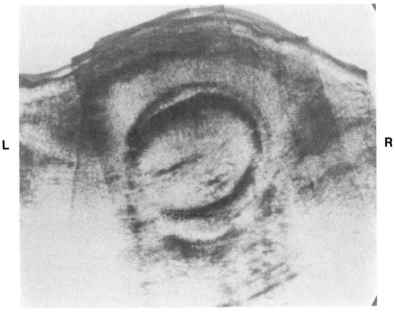

L   R

Fig. 4–16A. **Fetal head—Ida Clare** S+6

ANSWERS

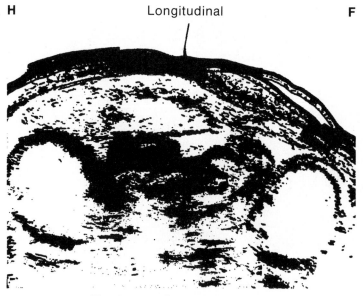

H   Longitudinal   F

Fig. 4–13B. Gemini—9 Months

If you diagnosed a two-headed baby, you're only half right. *Gemini* was happy to hear she would soon be eligible for lifetime membership in the Mothers of Twins Club. In the transverse echogram (Fig. 4–13A), a single falx echo is not clearly defined because the ultrasonic beam is traversing the fetal heads somewhat obliquely rather than in the exact biparietal plane. Shortly before delivery, a longitudinal examination (Fig. 4–13B) showed that the twins had done some moving around. One twin is now in the cephalic presentation, while the other is breech. Note the sharp line of the chorionic plate anteriorly.

The outcome for *Mrs. O'Hara* was less happy. Although the echogram (Fig. 4–14A) revealed a well-developed fetal body, no fetal head could be delineated in any of the sections. In addition, there was polyhydramnios. Look back and note the large clear space surrounding the fetal body. This finding is always suggestive of fetal abnormality. *Mrs. O'Hara's* first child was also anencephalic, a condition more common in children of Irish families. Anencephaly is also more common in the Sikhs of India. Figure 4–14B is a radiograph of the fetal head following delivery. Although the facial bones are intact, there is no real cranium. The baby died shortly after birth.

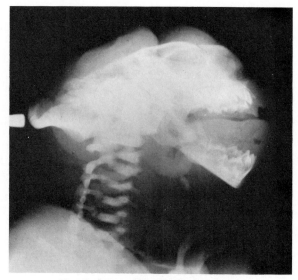

Fig. 4–14B. Mrs. O'Hara's baby

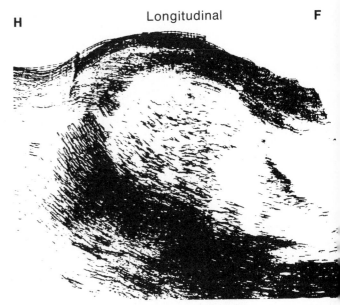

H   Longitudinal   F

Transverse (Fig. 4–15*A*) and longitudinal (Fig. 4–15*B*) examination of *Marvel's* uterus revealed it to be filled with many fine echoes, characteristic of a solid mass. No fetal parts were evident. On the basis of this echogram and markedly elevated human chorionic gonadotropin levels, a diagnosis of hydatidiform mole was made. The uterus was emptied.

Fig. 4–15B. **Marvel**

Fig. 4–16B. **Ida Clare**

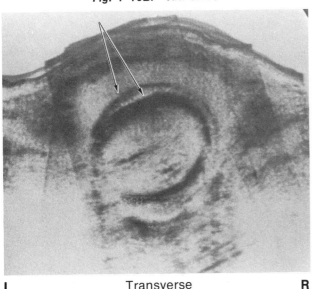

L   Transverse   R

Ida's worries were justified. The fetal head shows a coarsened "double" outline (arrows, Fig. 4–16*B*). This indicates marked edema, and is usually seen with fetal demise. A similar appearance may, however, be seen with diabetes or Rh isoimmunization. Other echographic signs of fetal death include poor definition of the falx echo; abnormal shape of the head; and "fluffy" outline of the head, thorax, or extremities. Failure of the fetus to move during the study and failure of the biparietal diameter to increase in successive studies also are suggestive of fetal death. One day after this study, Ida delivered a macerated fetus.

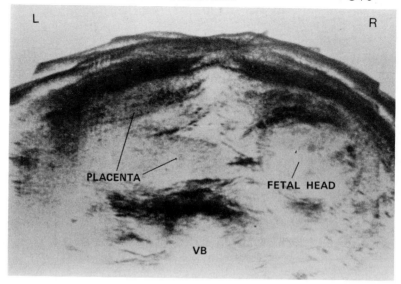

Fig. 4–17A.

AN UNUSUALLY LARGE PLACENTA

On this page you can examine transverse (Fig. 4–17A) and longitudinal (Fig. 4–17B) echograms of a large, boggy placenta extending both anteriorly and posteriorly. In this patient, the placenta covers more than 50 per cent of the internal surface of the uterus, and also the entire internal os. Large placentas are commonly seen in diabetics, in patients with Rh incompatibility and, of course, in multiple gestations.

Longitudinal L3

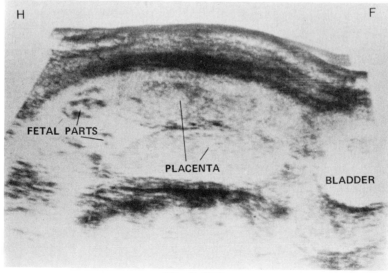

Fig. 4–17B.

THE LAST WORD

"But can't you tell me what *sex* it is?" say most mothers-to-be when the scan is completed. Usually we can't say, but every once in a while we're lucky. For instance:

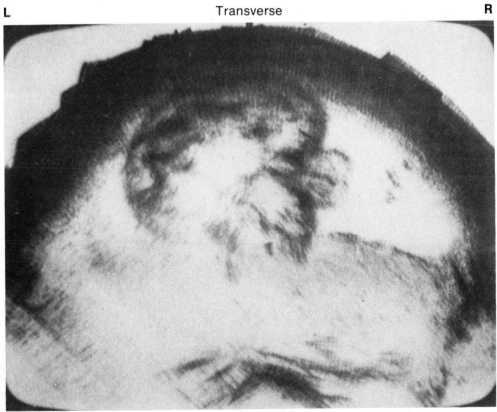

Fig. 4–18.   *Courtesy of Dr. Norman Swenson.*

It's a Boy!

USES OF ULTRASOUND IN GYNECOLOGY AND OBSTETRICS

GYNECOLOGY

1. IUCD localization

2. Pelvic mass work-up
   a. fluid-filled or solid
   b. relationship to uterus and adnexa

3. Pelvic abscess

OBSTETRICS

1. Confirmation of pregnancy when other tests are inconclusive or conflicting

2. Fetal gestational age

3. Fetal death

4. Multiple gestation

5. Fetal anomalies (hydrocephaly, anencephaly, large meningocele, hydrops, fetal ascites, etc.)

6. Placental location (previa, localization for amniocentesis)

7. Abruptio placentae

8. Hydramnios

9. Hydatidiform mole

CHAPTER 5

USES OF THE A-MODE

Instead of position-angle computers and storage scopes, the pioneers in diagnostic ultrasonography had only standard non-storage oscilloscopes, with a single horizontal baseline. Studies done with this type of display are known as A-mode (or amplitude mode) studies. Using this technique, the transducer is directed toward the area of interest. The electrical signal generated by returning echoes is displayed on the oscilloscope as a vertical deflection from the baseline. The height of this A-mode spike is proportional to the strength of the acoustic interface (thus, stronger interfaces produce spikes of greater amplitude). The machine is calibrated for the speed of sound in soft tissue, so that the spikes can be displayed at a certain distance along the baseline corresponding to the depth of the interface which produced them. When the beam strikes an interface between two tissues of differing acoustic density, an echo is returned (Fig. 5–1). The remainder of the beam continues to travel deeper into the tissues, striking other interfaces, and returning more echoes.

ACOUSTIC INTERFACE

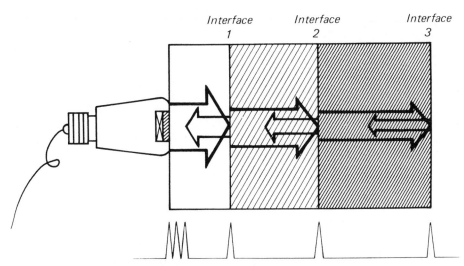

Fig. 5–1. A-mode recording. When the beam strikes an acoustic interface, the resulting echo is recorded as an A-mode spike on the oscilloscope. The position of the spike corresponds to the distance of the interface from the transducer.

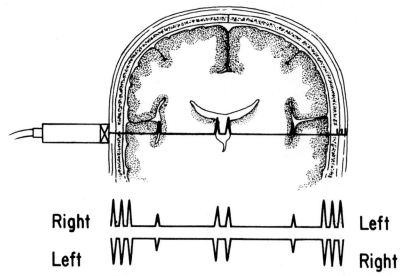

Right **Left**

Left **Right**

Fig. 5–2. Echoencephalogram. Echoes are recorded from the outer and inner tables of the skull, Sylvian fissures, and walls of the third ventricle. Two tracings are recorded on each picture: one obtained from the right side (top) and one obtained from the left side (bottom).

Echoencephalography

The primary use of the A-mode technique today is in echoencephalography. The ultrasonic beam is aimed through the thinnest portion of the temporal bone, just superoanterior to the pinna. (Yes, ultrasound *can* penetrate bone if the bone is very thin.) By directing the beam appropriately, echoes may be returned from the walls of the third ventricle, thus localizing its position relative to the inner tables of the skull on each side. The third ventricular echoes will be the strongest pair of spikes seen on the oscilloscope screen. In order to confirm results, the study is repeated with the transducer positioned on the opposite side of the skull. By convention, the study performed from the right side is photographed at the top of the picture, whereas the study performed from the left side is photographed beneath (Fig. 5–2).

Often, owing to multiple echoes from the air/skin (or transducer/skin), skin/skull, and skull/brain interfaces on each side, it may be difficult to determine just which echo actually represents the inner table. In order to obviate this problem, with its attendant difficulties in computing exactly where the midline should be, you may use the echograph itself to compute the theoretical position of the midline. If the third ventricular echoes match up in position with the theoretical midline, then we know that there is no midline shift.

THEORETICAL MIDLINE

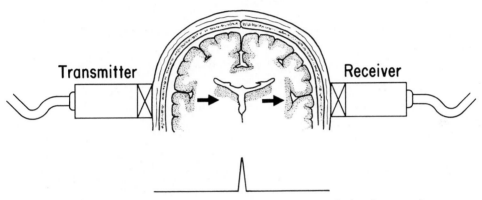

Fig. 5–3. Theoretical midline. Two transducers are used simultaneously, one as a transmitter and the other as a receiver. An A-mode spike is recorded at a point exactly halfway between the two transducers.

How is this theoretical midline determined? Instead of using one transducer as both transmitter and receiver (as is done with all other diagnostic studies), when determining the theoretical midline *two* transducers must be used simultaneously. One functions as a transmitter, the other as a receiver. With one transducer held to each temporal bone, the beam is then sent through the skull from one transducer and is received by the other. The distance the beam travels from one transducer face to the other is exactly the same as the distance the beam would travel if it had gone from one transducer face to the anatomic midline of the skull and then back to the same transducer. Therefore, an A-mode spike is recorded on the screen at this theoretical midline (Fig. 5–3). In the following studies, the theoretical midline determination is shown as the *middle* tracing.

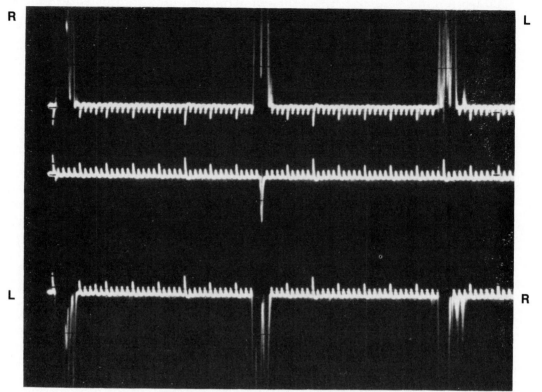

Fig. 5–4. Mel's echoencephalogram

LET'S SEE HOW YOU DO WITH A FEW PATIENTS

Mel Aze, 82, woke up this morning with right-sided weakness and some inability to express his thoughts clearly. You feel that his symptoms are due to a cerebrovascular accident, but want to rule out a subdural hematoma in view of a questionable history of trauma two weeks ago. Skull films (not shown) are entirely normal; however, the position of the pineal gland could not be seen well, so an echoencephalogram was obtained (Fig. 5–4).

ANSWER

Mel's echoencephalogram is normal. On both the right-to-left (top) and left-to-right (bottom) tracings a double-peaked echo is seen in the midline (the top of each peak is cut off the picture). This double peak is due to the small lateral dimension of the third ventricle; the spike representing the near wall does not return to the baseline before the spike representing the far wall takes off. This produces a wide-based M-shaped spike. The M-shaped spikes on both tracings line up with each other and also with the theoretical midline (middle tracing). Mel *did* have a stroke.

SOUND ADVICE: Does a normal echoencephalogram ("no midline shift") mean that there is no intracranial mass lesion? Not necessarily. Remember that the echoencephalogram only measures the position of the third ventricle. A mass lesion located far anteriorly or far posteriorly may not affect the position of the third ventricle. Similarly, bilateral lesions (such as multiple metastases or bilateral subdural hematomas) may cancel out each other's effects, and produce no midline shift.

PROBLEM

Claude Frogg, 43, South African high jumper turned novelist, has suffered from increasingly severe headaches during the past three months. Examination of his eyegrounds shows papilledema. Skull films (Fig. 5–5A) show no evidence of abnormality. The pineal gland was not calcified, however, so that the presence or absence of a midline shift could not be evaluated on the films. An echoencephalogram (Fig. 5–5B) was obtained.

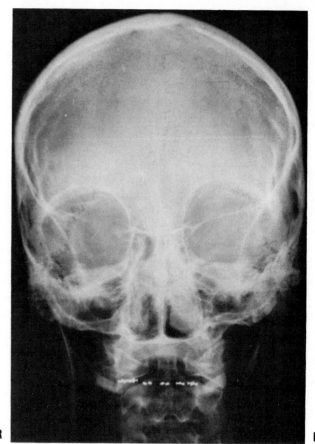

Fig. 5–5A. **Mr. Frogg's skull film**

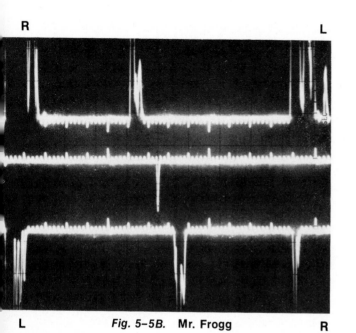

Fig. 5–5B. **Mr. Frogg**

ANSWER

Mr. Frogg has a shift of the midline to the right of approximately 11 mm. The theoretical midline is at 7.5 cm. The top tracing shows the midpoint of the M-complex to be at 6.4 cm., closer to the right side of the skull. The bottom tracing shows the midpoint of the midline complex to be at 8.6 cm., again closer to the right side of the skull. These measurements are accurate within 2 mm.

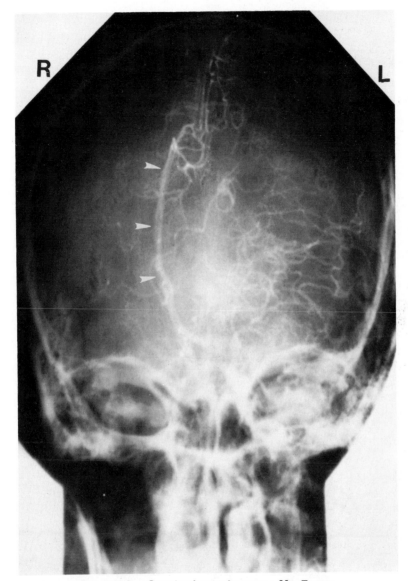

Fig. 5–5C. **Cerebral arteriogram — Mr. Frogg**

On the cerebral angiogram (Fig. 5–5C), there was a 15 mm. shift of the anterior cerebral artery (arrow) to the right, due to a temporal lobe glioblastoma. *How do you account for this apparent discrepancy in the amount of shift?*

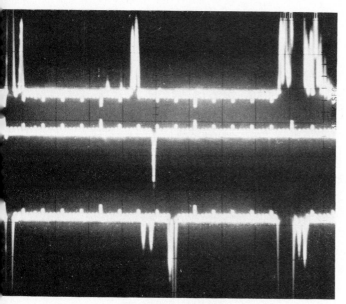

Fig. 5–6A.   Lionel

Lionel Schaft, who is 17 years old, was emulating the gymnastics of one of his heroes when he fell, striking his head. Although unconscious for approximately five minutes, Lionel is now alert (but somewhat sore). Your neurological exam shows no evidence of localizing signs. To be on the safe side, however, you obtain an echoencephalogram (Fig. 5–6A).

Donnie Brook, a 27-year-old local tough, suffered a collision with the large end of a cue stick approximately two weeks ago. He is brought to the Emergency Room by associates at 2 A.M. On examination, the right pupil is dilated and fixed, but there are no other localizing signs. The patient is grossly obtunded. Skull films (not shown) are normal.

THREE HEADS

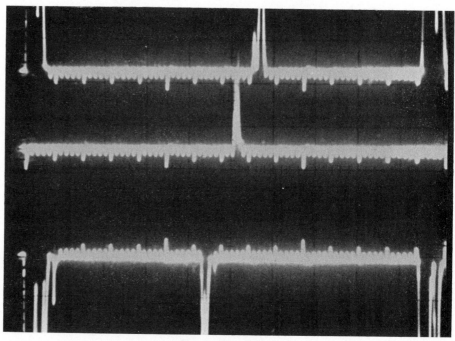

Fig. 5–7A.   Donnie

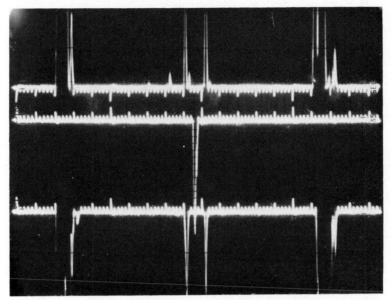

Fig. 5–8A. **Dr. Atrick**

Jerry Atrick, age 60, Nobel Laureate (physics), has been noted by friends to have sadly diminished mental capacity in the past year. His gait is also somewhat unusual. During routine physical examination, the patient was noted to evacuate his entire bladder contents.

ANSWER TO QUESTION ON PAGE 125: The echoencephalogram measures the degree of shift of the third ventricle from the midline. This may be greater or less than the shift of the more anteriorly located anterior cerebral artery.

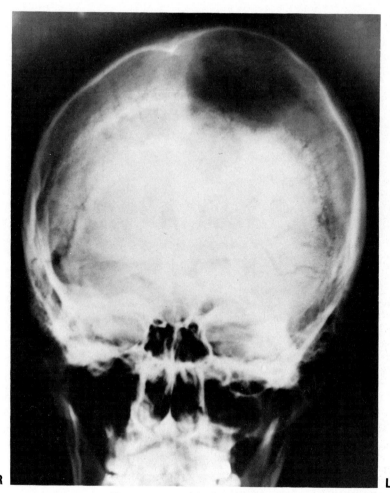

R L

Fig. 5–6B. Lionel's skull film

ANSWERS

Lionel's echogram (Fig. 5–6A) is certainly startling. It shows a shift to the right of approximately 10 mm. The skull films (Fig. 5–6B) are even more of a surprise. Note the marked asymmetry, with the left side of the calvarium enlarged when compared with the right. Pneumoencephalogram (not shown) revealed little cerebral tissue on the left. The entire left brain was replaced by a large porencephalic cyst, enlarging and thinning the cranium on that side. This is thought to be caused by intrauterine anoxia and subsequent maldevelopment. *Lionel*, with an IQ of 96, functioned just fine with his normal right cerebrum, which was squeezed into the smaller right side of his skull. His third ventricle actually *did* lie 10 mm. to the right of the midpoint between the outer tables of his skull. This is why the echoencephalographer must be cautious when attempting to evaluate asymmetrical skulls.

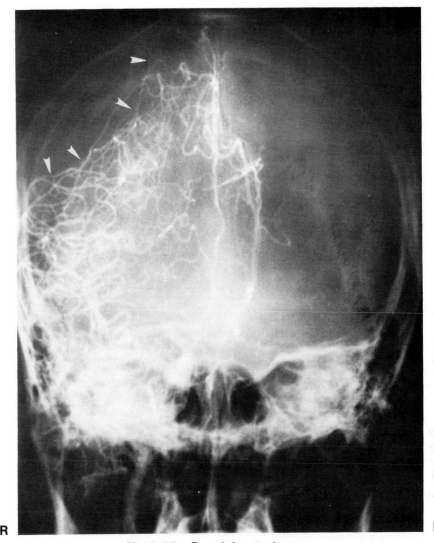

Fig. 5–7B. **Donnie's arteriogram**

Donnie's echoencephalogram reveals a shift to the left of approximately 10 mm. An emergency cerebral arteriogram (Fig. 5–7B) shows marked displacement of cortical vessels away from the inner table of the skull (arrows). (These vessels mark the outer surface of the brain, and ordinarily are seen just beneath the inner table.) The patient was immediately taken to surgery, where a large subdural hematoma was evacuated. In 10 days, *Donnie* was back in the pool hall.

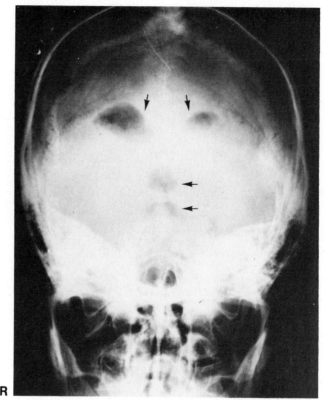

R   L

Courtesy of Dr. Marc Coel.

Fig. 5–8B. **Dr. Atrick's pneumoencephalogram**

ANSWERS — *Continued*

Dr. Atrick's third ventricle is in the midline, but the two walls are more separated from each other than usual: 12 mm., to be exact. Pneumoencephalogram (Fig. 5–8B) shows generalized ventricular enlargement (arrows) without widening of the sulci.

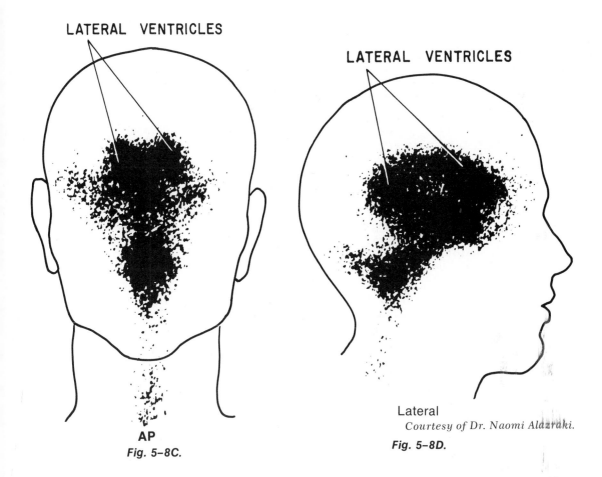

LATERAL VENTRICLES

LATERAL VENTRICLES

AP

Fig. 5–8C.

Lateral

Courtesy of Dr. Naomi Alazraki.

Fig. 5–8D.

Isotope cisternogram (Figs. 5–8C and 5–8D) reveals accumulation of the isotope in the basal cisterns and the ventricles 24 hours after injection into the lumbar subarachnoid space. There is no isotope over the cerebral convexities, however. These findings are characteristic of normal pressure hydrocephalus, a disease in which normal absorption of cerebrospinal fluid by the arachnoid villi does not take place. The classical triad seen clinically includes ataxia, dementia, and incontinence. Ten days after a ventriculoperitoneal shunt was installed, *Dr. Atrick* was again writing indecipherable equations.

> NOTE: In some centers, ultrasound is also used to measure the size of the lateral ventricles. This is technically more difficult than measurement of the size and position of the third ventricle.

Ophthalmic Studies

The A-mode technique may be used for other purposes as well. In ophthalmology, the acoustically empty vitreous allows recognition of abnormalities of the interior of the globe, such as intraocular foreign bodies, retinal detachments and tumors. Axial length (cornea–retina) may also be accurately determined using this method. It is particularly useful in evaluating eyes in which clouding or hemorrhage prevents satisfactory visualization of internal structure. Special high-frequency transducers are used for these studies. These transducers provide high resolution of soft tissue detail at the expense of diminished depth penetration, and thus are ideal for a superficially located organ such as the eye. The transducer may be placed on the eyelid (using a connecting medium such as a bubble-free gel) or directly on the anesthetized cornea.

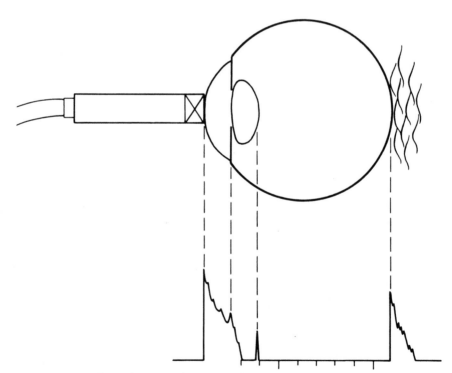

Fig. 5–9. **A-mode ophthalmic echogram. The vitreous is echo-free.**

A-mode study characteristically shows a complex of multiple echoes from the anterior chamber of the eye and the lens. Sometimes the echo from the posterior surface of the lens is separable from the remainder of the anterior complex (Fig. 5–9). Under normal circumstances, no echoes are seen within the interior of the globe (as the sound passes without interference through the homogeneous vitreous). The posterior surface of the globe and orbital structures produce another wide complex of echoes, gradually diminishing in strength.

It is also possible (using special ophthalmic scanners) to perform B-mode studies of the eye. Two types of ophthalmic B-scanners are currently in use. They both provide additional structural information about intraocular and retrobulbar pathology; one type also gives a more detailed picture of the anterior chamber.

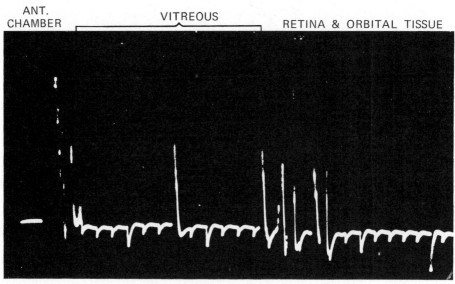

| ANT. CHAMBER | VITREOUS | RETINA & ORBITAL TISSUE |

Fig. 5–10A. **Ophthalmic study. J. W. Berdon**

PROBLEM

J. Whiteman Berdon, who is 53 years old, is the newly appointed U. S. Consul to a small, divided country. While he was inspecting his quarters, a commotion in the Consulate courtyard caused him to run to the window. Unfortunately, at this point a satchel charge detonated against the wall, and the Consulate windows imploded. *J. W.* is one of 26 injured persons brought to your small hospital. He has multiple facial lacerations, with soft tissue swelling particularly marked about the right eye. Facial films (not shown) confirm the soft tissue swelling, but there is no fracture and no visible foreign body. After prying apart the lids, you attempt to examine the eye. There is severe disruption of the lens, however, which prevents you from seeing into the vitreous. A-mode echogram (Fig. 5–10A) was done through the closed lid.

HINT: Although glass is ordinarily visible on x-ray, a small fragment may easily be missed, particularly when a large amount of soft tissue swelling is present.

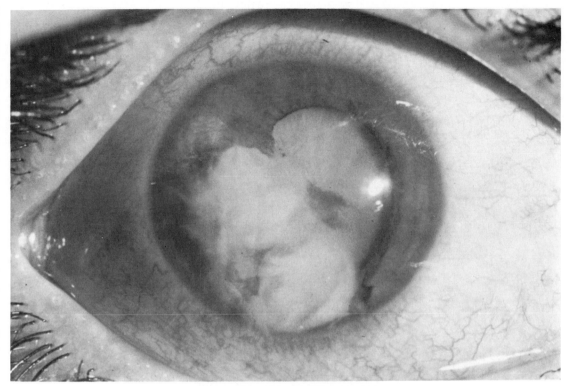

Fig. 5–10B. **Traumatic cataract**

ANSWER

The echogram (Fig. 5–10A) shows a single tall spike in the otherwise empty vitreous. When the patient moved his eye, then brought it back to its original direction, the position of the spike changed. This is characteristic of a foreign body floating within the vitreous.

J. W. was evacuated to the continental U.S., where the traumatic cataract (Fig. 5–10B) was removed, allowing him to regain his vision. Two weeks later, examination of the vitreous confirmed the presence of a small fragment of glass floating within. This fragment did not require removal since it is inert. (It *would* be necessary to remove a noninert foreign body, such as copper or iron.)

The A-mode echogram is particularly valuable in the preoperative evaluation of metallic foreign bodies. Once the foreign body is localized with ultrasound, a magnetic field is generated near the eye through the use of an ophthalmic electromagnet. If the A-mode spike of the foreign body moves when the magnet is turned on, the surgeon knows that the fragment is magnetic. This becomes vitally important during surgery for removal of the fragment. After making the incision into the eye, the surgeon can use the magnet to move the fragment into position for removal.

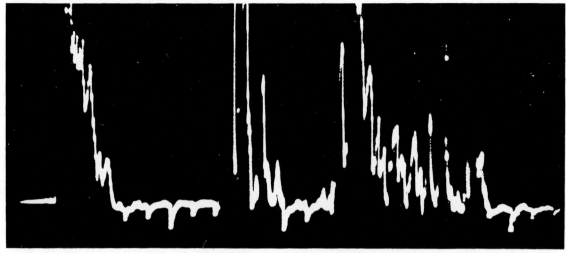

Fig. 5–11A. **Caesar—A-mode**

ANT. CHAMBER   TUMOR   ORBITAL TISSUE

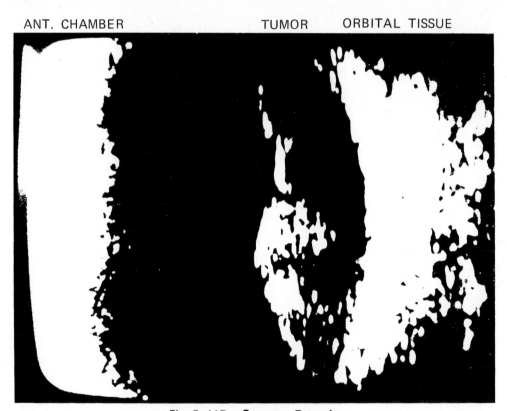

Fig. 5–11B. **Caesar—B-mode**

PROBLEM

Caesar Pallas, a 42-year-old shill, comes to you complaining of a "curtain" entering the line of sight of his left eye. You note that his sclerae are slightly icteric, but Caesar can't tell you how long they have been that way. He denies any abnormal coloration of urine or stool but does confess to a 10 pound weight loss over the past three months. Examination of the fundus reveals a mass just superior to the optic nerve. Both A-mode (Fig. 5–11A) and B-mode (Fig. 5–11B) echograms were obtained to provide some information as to the internal structure of the mass.

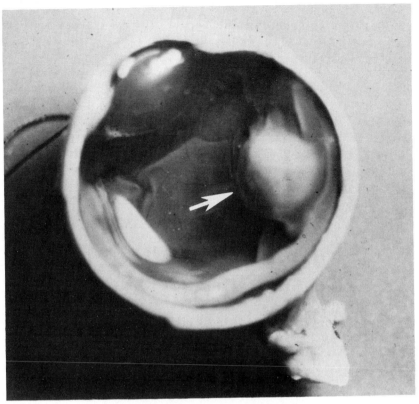

Fig. 5-11C. **Melanoma, enucleated eye**

ANSWER

Both studies reveal a cluster of weak and strong echoes returning from the mass. This appearance is characteristic of a solid lesion. *Caesar's* complaint of a "curtain" over his vision is caused by detachment of the overlying retina by the mass. Further workup confirms your suspicion of malignant melanoma, metastatic to the liver. In view of the known metastatic disease, enucleation is not indicated. Melanoma is the most common primary eye tumor in adults. Figure 5-11C shows the enucleated specimen from another patient.

> TEACHING POINT: One great value of both A-mode and B-mode ophthalmic ultrasound is the ability to distinguish between a simple retinal detachment and a solid detachment (one caused by an underlying mass). The surgeon can then be guided toward the appropriate operation: for the simple retinal detachment, a vision-restoring procedure; for the solid detachment, a life-saving enucleation.

Pleural Studies

The A-mode technique may also be used in the localization of pleural effusions and in the differentiation of pleural fluid from pleural thickening. When the transducer is placed on the normal thorax, there is unsatisfactory penetration of the ultrasonic beam because of reflection from the air-containing lung. If a pleural effusion is present, however, the beam will traverse the fluid, and an echo-free space may be seen on the A-mode study (Fig. 5–12). This technique is particularly useful when localizing small loculated effusions for thoracentesis. The A-mode unit is portable, and the examination can be done at the patient's bedside. If the patient can be brought to the Ultrasound Department, even better delineation of effusions can be obtained using the B-scanner.

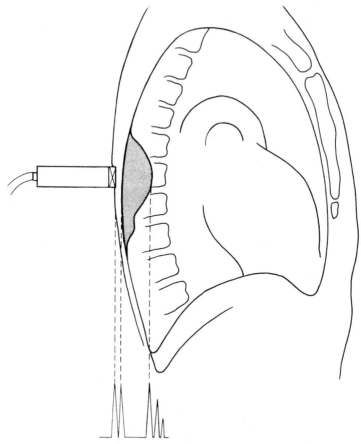

Fig. 5–12. **Loculated pleural effusion. The A-mode echogram shows an echo-free space corresponding to the location and size of the effusion.**

PROBLEM

Philbert Grove, a California almond grower who is 49 years old, spent several weeks in the hospital with a right lower lobe abscess (post-aspiration) and associated empyema. Now he is recovering, but chest films (Fig. 5–13A) still show a large area of "pleural thickening" (or is it loculated purulent fluid?) in his right posterior hemithorax. An attempt at thoracentesis was unsuccessful, so an echogram (Fig. 5–13A) was requested to determine the nature of the mass.

P 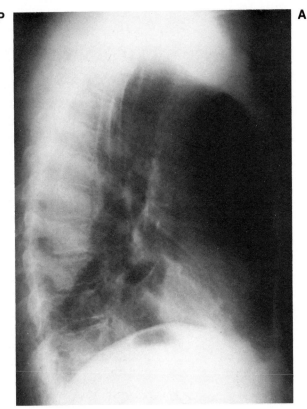 A

Fig. 5–13A. **Mr. Grove—Lateral chest film**

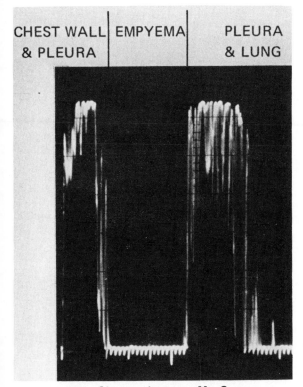

CHEST WALL | EMPYEMA | PLEURA
& PLEURA | | & LUNG

Fig. 5–13B. **Chest echogram. Mr. Grove**

ANSWER

The A-mode transducer was placed in the right sixth interspace posteriorly, just medial to the scapula. An echo-free area measuring approximately 4 cm. in depth was identified (Fig. 5–13B). This appearance is characteristic of fluid. (Solid pleural thickening would have shown multiple echoes rather than an echo-free space). The skin site was marked with a wax pencil, and repeat thoracentesis (using a larger-bore needle) was performed. Approximately 10 cc. of thick purulent fluid was withdrawn. Following this, a chest tube was inserted and free flow of fluid was obtained. *Mr. Grove's* recovery was uneventful.

Aspirations and Biopsies

A-mode may also be useful during the actual performance of a thoracentesis, renal cyst puncture or organ biopsy. A special transducer with a central hole ("aspiration" or "biopsy" transducer) is used (Fig. 5–14). The area of interest is first localized with B-mode, its depth from the skin surface is measured on the scan, and the overlying skin surface is marked. The patient is prepped and draped, and local anesthetic is injected. Then the sterile aspiration transducer is placed on the skin mark and directed toward the area of interest. When the desired complex of echoes appears on the screen (an echo-free space in the case of a pleural effusion, for instance), the needle is inserted through the central hole until its tip (represented by a strong echo) can be seen within the previously echo-free space. The fluid is then withdrawn, and as this happens the echo-free space on the oscilloscope screen can be seen to become progressively smaller.

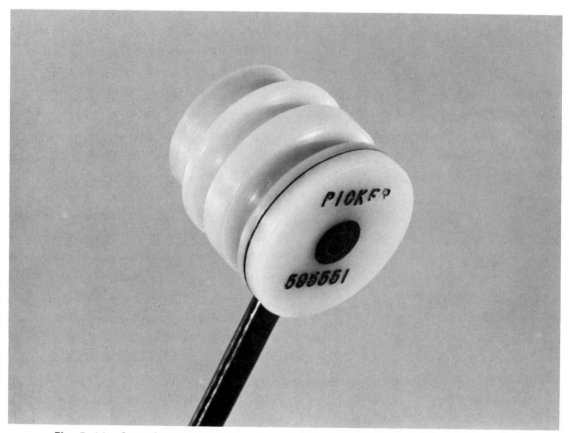

Fig. 5–14. **A-mode aspiration transducer. Note central hole for passage of the needle. B-mode aspiration transducers are also available.**

SUMMARY

1. The most frequent use of A-mode is in the determination of the position of the third ventricle (echoencephalogram). Intracranial lesions that do not displace the third ventricle from the midline will not be identified by this technique.

2. A-mode examination of the eye is particularly useful in determining axial length of the globe, and also in searching for intraocular foreign bodies. B-mode examination allows more precise definition of intraocular and retrobulbar masses.

3. A-mode is helpful in identifying and localizing pleural effusions. Differentiation between pleural fluid and pleural thickening may be made.

4. A special aspiration transducer may be used for ultrasound control during thoracentesis, renal cyst puncture, or renal biopsy.

CHAPTER 6

ECHOCARDIOGRAPHY

Echocardiography is one of the most rapidly expanding applications of diagnostic ultrasound. Using ultrasound, the physician can gain an accurate picture of cardiac valve and chamber *motion*, and also of the anatomy of the cardiac structures.

At present, most echocardiography is performed with a single transducer. Units are available, however, in which a linear array of several transducers is used to produce a picture of a single plane of the heart. These pictures look much like B-mode scans with one important difference: the entire section can be seen instantaneously (rather than being "built up" by multiple passes of the scanning transducer), and in motion.

This chapter will concentrate on single-transducer echocardiography.

When performing echocardiograms, the M-mode (*motion*) format is used. With this type of recording, a picture can be obtained showing the position of moving structures over a period of several seconds. The structures are represented by dots (as in B-mode) rather than by A-mode spikes. Unlike B-mode, however, the baseline is moved across the screen over a period of several seconds (Fig. 6–1). The picture thus produced shows the position of the cardiac structures (as represented by coalescent dots) for the previous several seconds. If any of the structures being recorded are changing position, their movement toward or away from the transducer will be accurately identified (Fig. 6–2).

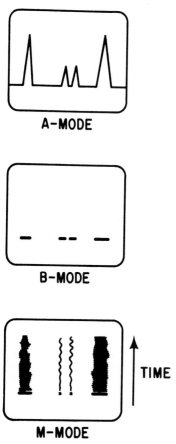

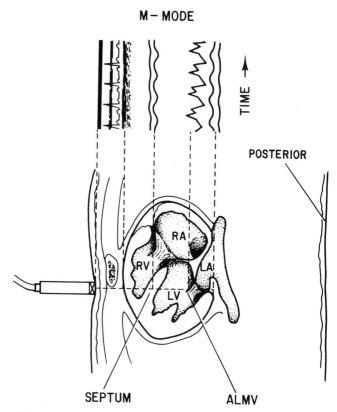

Fig. 6–1. In M-mode the echoes are represented as dots, which are moved across the screen over a period of several seconds. Due to the relatively slow sweep, the dots coalesce and are recorded as lines. Motion of the structures toward and away from the transducer may be depicted this way.

Fig. 6–2. Transverse section of the heart with corresponding M-mode trace. The chest wall is to the left of the picture.

The M-mode picture may be recorded in several ways: the picture on the screen may be photographed on Polaroid film or recorded on heat-sensitive paper; or a strip-chart recorder (with light-sensitive paper) may be used. This latter recording system has many advantages and is the method of choice in centers doing a large volume of echocardiography.

The completed echocardiographic tracing is not read from bottom to top, but is turned clockwise 90 degrees and read from left to right (Fig. 6–3). This convention was adopted so that the electrocardiographic tracing, which is usually superimposed along one side of the strip, can also be read in the usual left to right manner.

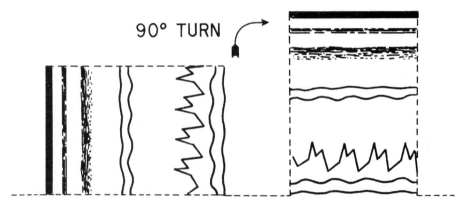

Fig. 6–3. The echocardiographic tracing is read from left to right. Thus, the tracing is turned so that chest wall is at the top of the picture, rather than to the left.

In order to appreciate fully the echocardiographic tracing, an accurate understanding of cardiac anatomy is essential. Figure 6–4 shows a longitudinal section extending from the aortic root to the cardiac apex. This is the path along which the ultrasonic transducer is sequentially directed for the basic echocardiographic examination.

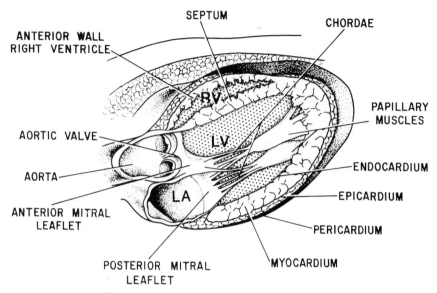

Fig. 6–4. **Longitudinal view of the heart.**

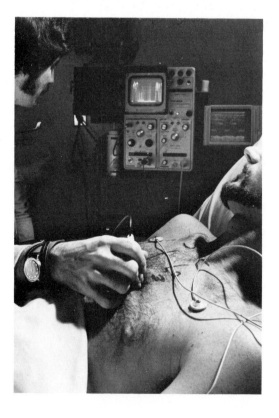

The transducer (no longer attached to the rigid arm that is necessary for B-mode studies) is generally placed in the fourth interspace just to the left of the sternum (Fig. 6–5). This allows the examiner to aim the beam through the skin, muscle, and mediastinal tissues before contacting the cardiac structures. If the transducer is placed too laterally, the beam will strike the air-filled lung and be almost completely reflected without striking the heart.

Fig. 6–5. **Sonographer performing echocardiogram. The transducer is in the 4th intercostal space, left of the sternum. The oscilloscope shows the A-mode trace. The corresponding M-mode trace (turned 90°) is seen on the screen to the right. Electrocardiographic leads are in place.**

With the transducer in this position, the examiner can then angle the instrument, directing the beam superomedially to strike the aortic root or inferolaterally to delineate the cardiac apex. Between these two positions, the mitral valve may be identified. It is apparent that the direction in which the examiner aims the transducer must depend upon the anatomy of the individual patient. For example, the beam will traverse a more horizontal arc in a short, fat patient, and a more vertical arc in a tall, thin patient (Figs. 6–6A and 6–6B).

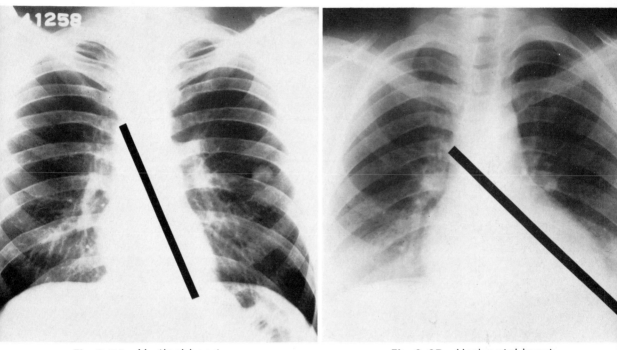

Fig. 6–6A. Vertical heart   *Fig. 6–6B.* Horizontal heart

The bar shows the direction in which the transducer must be directed to produce a satisfactory echocardiogram.

By the way, did you notice the small collection of air beneath the right hemidiaphragm in the patient with the horizontal heart? This patient had recently undergone abdominal surgery.

The patient with the vertical heart has a coin lesion in his left midlung field, seen overlying the interspace between the third and fourth anterior ribs. At surgery, it proved to be a bronchogenic carcinoma.

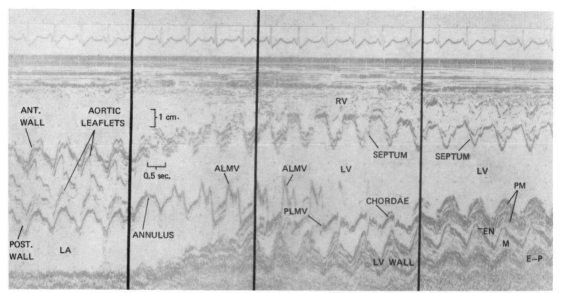

Fig. 6-7. Echocardiogram. The nonmoving echoes anteriorly arise from the chest wall. This tracing has been divided into four sections for discussion.

Figure 6–7 shows an echocardiogram that was obtained as the transducer was directed in an arc from the aortic root (left) to the cardiac apex (right). Figure 6–8 shows the arc through which the transducer must be directed to produce such a picture.

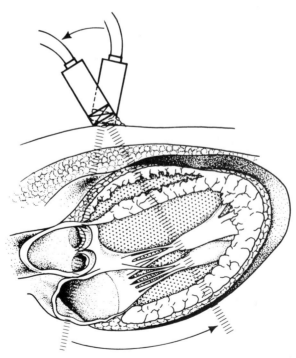

Fig. 6-8. The transducer must be directed in an arc from the aortic root to the cardiac apex (or vice versa) in order to obtain a complete tracing such as the one in Figure 6–7.

When the transducer is aimed superomedially (Fig. 6–9A), the beam traverses the aortic root. The anterior and posterior walls of the root (Fig. 6–9B) are seen as strong lines moving in the same direction at the same time. During systole (identified by the electrocardiogram at the top of the picture), the walls of the aortic root move anteriorly, or toward the transducer. During diastole, the aortic root moves posteriorly. This motion reflects the motion of the entire heart anteriorly with ventricular contraction and posteriorly with ventricular relaxation.

Within the walls of the aortic root, the aortic leaflets (Figs. 6–9B and 6–9C) can be seen, opening to produce a boxlike pattern during systole. Behind the aortic root is the left atrial cavity (LA).

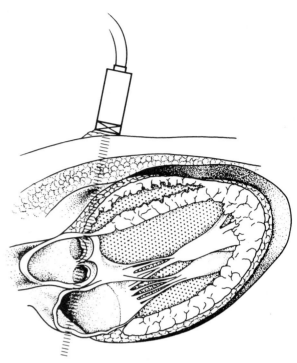

Fig. 6–9A. The transducer is directed toward the aortic root and left atrium.

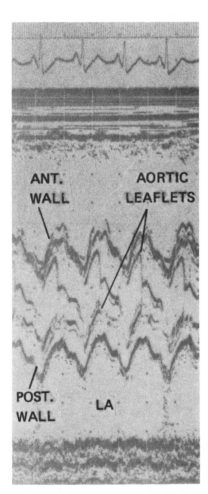

Fig. 6–9B. Aortic root and left atrium (LA). The aortic leaflets are open during systole, producing a parallelogram configuration.

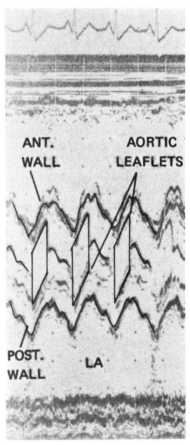

Fig. 6–9C. Aortic leaflets enhanced. The anterior side of the parallelogram is probably produced by the right coronary leaflet. The posterior tracing is produced by the noncoronary leaflet.

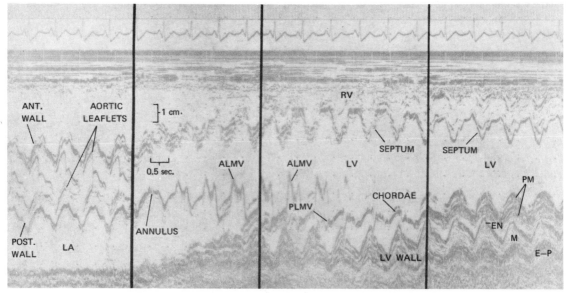

ANT. WALL · AORTIC LEAFLETS ·]1 cm. · RV · SEPTUM · SEPTUM · LV · ALMV · ALMV · LV · PM · 0.5 sec. · CHORDAE · EN · PLMV · M · POST. WALL · LA · ANNULUS · LV WALL · E–P

Echocardiogram. Sweep from aortic root to cardiac apex.

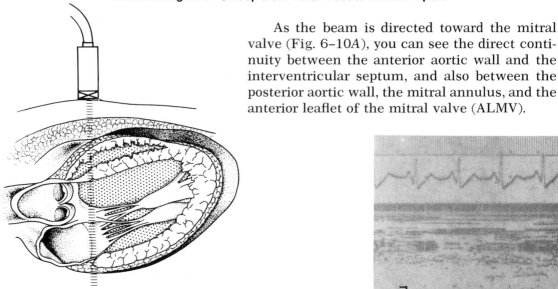

As the beam is directed toward the mitral valve (Fig. 6–10A), you can see the direct continuity between the anterior aortic wall and the interventricular septum, and also between the posterior aortic wall, the mitral annulus, and the anterior leaflet of the mitral valve (ALMV).

Fig. 6–10A. **The transducer is directed toward the anterior leaflet of the mitral valve. Note the continuity of the valve with the posterior wall of the aortic root.**

The anterior mitral leaflet (Fig. 6–10B) has a characteristic M-shaped pattern during diastole. The leaflet opens rapidly (moving anteriorly) at the onset of diastole, and then becomes partially closed (posterior motion) by the end of the rapid filling phase. With atrial systole, the leaflet re-opens, returning to the closed position by the onset of ventricular systole. During systole, the leaflet moves slightly anteriorly (passively), owing to the anterior motion of the entire heart with systole.

Fig. 6–10B. **Anterior mitral leaflet (ALMV). The interventricular septum is seen anteriorly. Septal motion cannot be evaluated at this level because of proximity to the aortic root, whose motion may be influenced by the septum.**

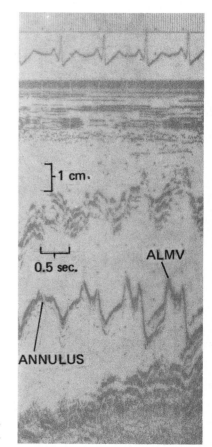

]1 cm.

0.5 sec. · ALMV

ANNULUS

Various points on the echo pattern of the anterior mitral leaflet have been labeled, by convention, A through F (Fig. 6–11A). The leaflet is completely closed (most posterior) at point C, and with ventricular systole gradually moves anteriorly to point D. With diastole, the leaflet then opens as blood rapidly flows from the left atrium into the left ventricle. Maximum leaflet opening is at point E. Following this initial rapid left ventricular filling, the leaflets partially close to point F. With atrial systole, the leaflets reopen to point A, then begin to close again during atrial relaxation. Ventricular systole occurs at point B, completing valve closure.

The initial diastolic closing velocity of the anterior mitral leaflet (E-F slope, see far right complex, Figure 6–11A) is an important indicator of the rate of blood flow from the left atrium into the left ventricle. The normal closing velocity is at least 60 mm./sec. and usually greater than 80 mm./sec. The E-F slope is reduced in patients with a reduced rate of left ventricular filling, such as patients with diminished compliance. Rates of less than 35 mm./sec. are characteristic of patients with hemodynamically significant mitral stenosis (Fig. 6–11B).

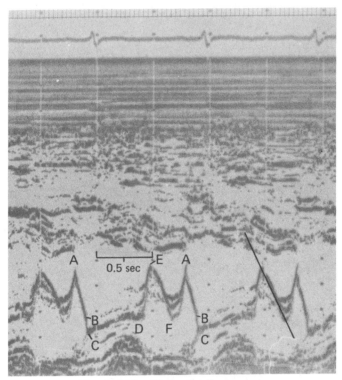

Fig. 6–11A. Normal mitral valve

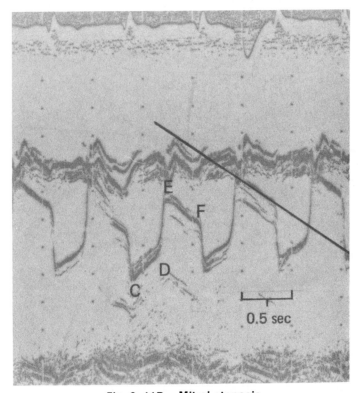

Fig. 6–11B. Mitral stenosis

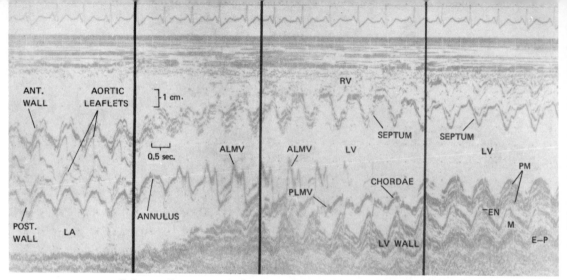

Echocardiogram. Sweep from aortic root to cardiac apex.

As the beam is directed more infero-laterally (Fig. 6–12A), the posterior mitral leaflet (PLMV) comes into view (Fig. 6–12B). This leaflet has a motion that is a small mirror image of the motion of the anterior mitral leaflet. (Anatomically, the posterior mitral leaflet actually *is* smaller than the anterior leaflet.) Just behind the posterior mitral leaflet is the posterior left ventricular wall. With each contraction, the diameter of the left ventricle decreases as the interventricular septum and the posterior left ventricular wall approach each other. The right ventricular cavity (RV) is poorly delineated in this tracing.

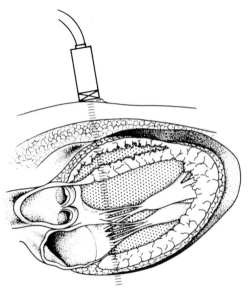

Fig. 6–12A. The transducer is directed at both the anterior and posterior leaflets of the mitral valve. It also traverses the left ventricular posterior wall.

When the transducer is aimed even more inferolaterally (right portion of Figure 6–12B) the anterior mitral leaflet is no longer visible. Finally, the posterior mitral leaflet also disappears. Instead of the typical M-shaped motion, we see only slight motion anteriorly during systole and posteriorly during diastole. This is the point at which the posterior mitral leaflet attaches to its chordae tendineae. Sometimes chordae tendineae attaching to the anterior mitral leaflet may also be seen.

Fig. 6–12B. Anterior (ALMV) and posterior (PLMV) mitral leaflets. As the transducer is directed more toward the apex (right side of picture), some chordae tendineae are seen. Note the opposing motion of the interventricular septum and the posterior left ventricular wall. This is a good position for evaluation of left ventricular size and function.

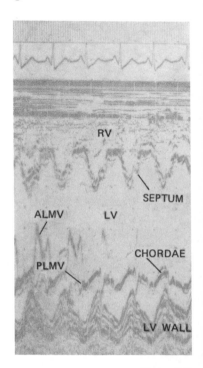

When the transducer is aimed deep into the apex of the left ventricle (Fig. 6–13A), the papillary muscle may be recorded lying anterior to the endocardium of the left ventricle. Note the smooth transition from posterior mitral leaflet to chordae tendineae to papillary muscle.

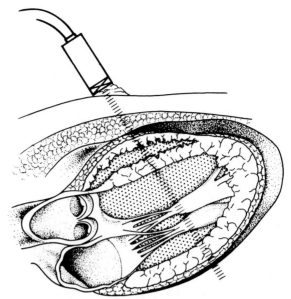

Fig. 6–13A. The transducer is directed into the left ventricular cavity.

In Figure 6–13B, the endocardium (EN) is represented by a fine line moving anteriorly with ventricular systole. Behind this, a series of fine lines represent the muscular fibers of the myocardium (M). The darkest, most posterior moving line is the epicardium–pericardium (E-P).

Note that the motion of the epipericardium is less than that of the endocardium during systole. This makes sense if you think of the heart as a bag with an outer surface (pericardium) and an inner lining (endocardium). As the spherical outer surface becomes smaller (contraction), the inner lining is thrown into folds.

The epicardium and pericardium are normally closely apposed. A clear separation between the two structures may be seen in patients with pericardial effusion.

It is important to be familiar with these normal patterns of cardiac structures so that abnormal patterns may be recognized.

Fig. 6–13B. Left ventricular cavity. The papillary muscle (PM) lies anterior to the LV wall. This position is too near the apex for evaluation of left ventricular size and function.

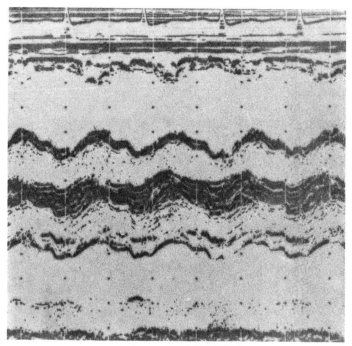

Fig. 6–14A. Don's aortic root

Donald Corleone, 62, importer, experienced pain associated with transient loss of consciousness while lifting a crate of olive oil this morning. He now recalls a similar episode about five weeks ago while carrying some groceries up the stairs. During your examination, you detect a loud, harsh systolic ejection murmur.

FOUR PATIENTS WITH SYSTOLIC MURMURS

Art Decco is a 31-year-old interior designer who has no real complaints. He thought it was just "time for a checkup." His physical examination is entirely normal with the exception of a mid-systolic murmur in the second left intercostal space and fixed splitting of the second heart sound. Art tells you that he's had that murmur since childhood and never worried about it since it never seemed to cause any trouble. He is flattered by your interest, however, and is agreeable to having an echocardiogram, since you assure him it's perfectly painless.

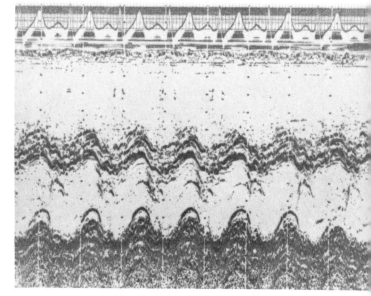

Fig. 6–15A. Art's left ventricle

Maida Bundle, a 28-year-old stockbroker, has noticed that occasionally her heart "flutters," so she comes to you for an examination. Her past history is unremarkable and her physical exam is entirely normal except for a Grade II late systolic murmur. You feel that this is probably a functional murmur, but obtain an echocardiogram just to be on the safe side.

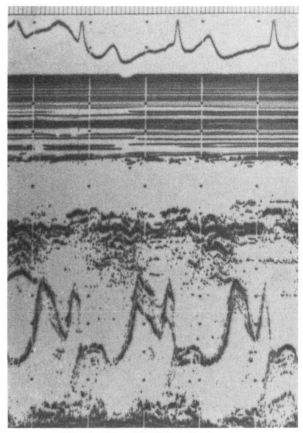

Fig. 6–16A. **Maida's mitral valve**

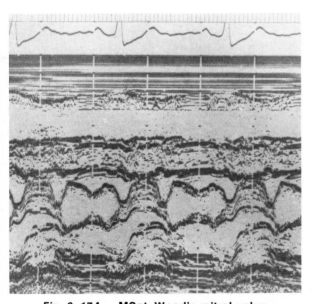

Fig. 6–17A. **MSgt. Wood's mitral valve**

Bellew Wood, 56, MSgt, USMC, Ret. (brother of Birnam Wood, pg. 73), has recently noted some chest pain and dyspnea while shooting baskets with his grandson. In addition, he tells you, he has had two or three episodes of "dizziness" within the past six months. On auscultation, you hear a systolic ejection murmur along the left sternal border.

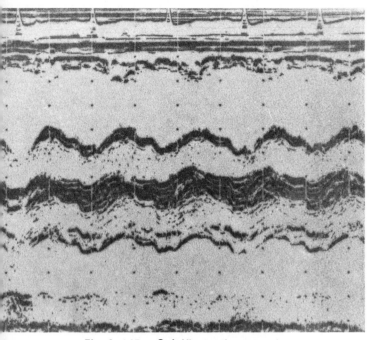

Fig. 6–14B. Calcific aortic stenosis

Don's echogram (Fig. 6–14B) shows findings typical of aortic stenosis. The leaflets are so thickened and calcified that they appear as a mass of dense echoes lying within the aortic root. No boxlike pattern of systolic opening can be identified in this tracing. (In patients with less involvement, diminished opening excursion of the leaflets can usually be identified.) *Chest pain and syncopal episodes are ominous findings in a patient with aortic stenosis.* Fortunately, *Don* did very well following surgical replacement of his damaged valve.

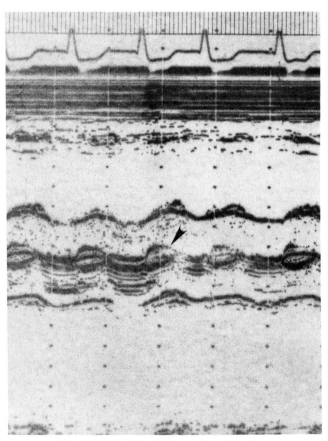

Fig. 6–14C. Another aortic stenosis

Figure 6–14C shows the aortic root tracing in another patient with severe aortic stenosis. Only slight systolic opening motion of the leaflets can be seen (arrow). This patient had concomitant mitral stenosis and insufficiency causing left atrial enlargement. Note the markedly enlarged left atrium just posterior to the aortic root (compare with Figure 6–14B). In a person of average size, the left atrial diameter usually does not exceed 4 cm. during atrial diastole.

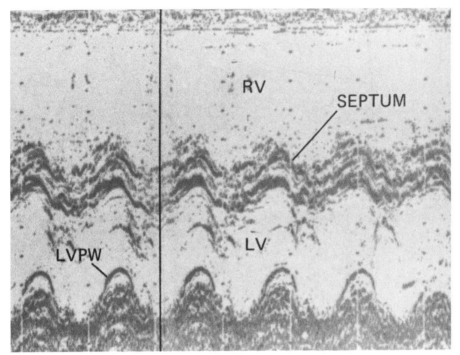

Fig. 6–15B. **Paradoxical septal motion**

ANSWERS—*Continued*

Art's aortic and mitral valves (not shown) looked perfectly normal on the echocardiogram. On the left ventricular tracing (Fig. 6–15B), however, two things are apparent. The right ventricle is enlarged (> 2.3 cm.) and the interventricular septum moves paradoxically; that is, instead of moving *toward* the left ventricular posterior wall during systole (posterior motion), the septum actually moves *away* (anterior motion). (Look at the motion of the septum and the left ventricular wall just following the vertical line dropped from the "R" wave of the electrocardiogram; the septum should move posteriorly at this point.) These two findings are characteristically found in right ventricular volume overload from any cause. As you probably suspected, Art had an atrial septal defect.

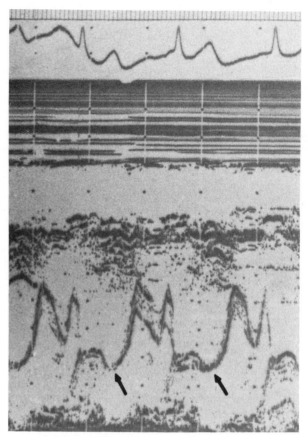

Fig. 6–16B. **Late systolic prolapse**

ANSWERS—*Continued*

Before you have a chance to discuss the study with the echocardiographer, your resident also listens to *Maida's* heart. In addition to the late systolic murmur, she hears a mid-systolic "click." Review of the echocardiographic tracing confirms your clinical diagnosis of late systolic prolapse of the mitral leaflet ("click-murmur syndrome"). Dur-

ing systole, both mitral leaflets ordinarily move slightly anteriorly, reflecting the motion of the mitral annulus. On *Maida's* tracing (Fig. 6–16B), the leaflets begin to move anteriorly during systole, but during the latter half of systole they suddenly drop posteriorly (arrows), reflecting prolapse into the left atrium. (The leaflets are closely apposed during systole and appear as a single line on most of the tracing.)

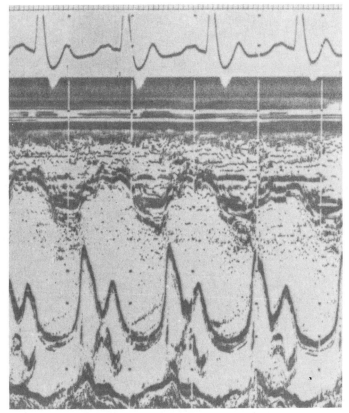

Fig. 6–16C. **Holosystolic prolapse**

ANSWERS – *Continued*

The echocardiographic findings with prolapsing mitral leaflet are somewhat variable. In some patients, the leaflets may prolapse during all of systole ("hammocking," Fig. 6–16C). The finding may be intermittent (as the murmur may also be). Or provocative measures, such as exercise or amyl nitrite inhalation, may be required to demonstrate the typical finding. Sometimes, only the posterior leaflet is seen to prolapse, whereas the anterior leaflet moves normally. It is important to make this diagnosis, because these patients have a higher than normal incidence of cardiac arrhythmias and of bacterial endocarditis.

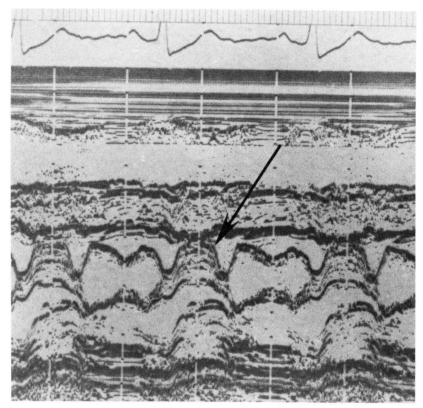

Fig. 6–17B.   **Idiopathic hypertrophic subaortic stenosis**

ANSWERS—*Continued*

MSgt. Wood has idiopathic hypertrophic subaortic stenosis (IHSS). The abnormality on this tracing is the unusual anterior motion (Fig. 6–17B) of the anterior mitral leaflet during systole (arrow). (Compare with Figure 6–16C, mitral valve prolapse, in which the mitral valve shows posterior "hammocking" during systole.) This systolic anterior motion (SAM) of the anterior mitral leaflet is characteristic of IHSS. Note also the diminished closing velocity (E-F slope) of the anterior mitral leaflet. This latter finding is common in patients with IHSS and is due to decreased left ventricular compliance.

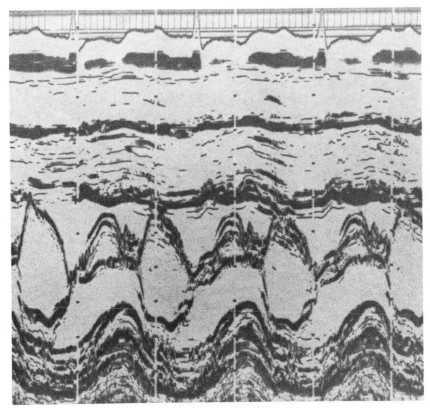

Fig. 6–17C. **Another IHSS**

ANSWERS – *Continued*

On further examination of *MSgt. Wood's* tracing, you can see that the interventricular septum is somewhat thick (> 1.2 cm.) and shows very little motion during systole. This finding is also characteristic of IHSS and, in fact, the disease is sometimes known as "asymmetrical septal hypertrophy" (ASH) because the mid and upper portions of the septum are markedly hypertrophied compared to the normal thickness of the posterior left ventricular wall. Figure 6–17C is a tracing from another patient with IHSS and similar echocardiographic findings. Note the markedly thickened, almost immobile septum, the prominent SAM, and the diminished mitral E-F slope (the "A" wave is not seen as a separate excursion in this tracing). Many observers feel that systolic anterior motion of the anterior mitral leaflet is due to a Venturi effect of blood rushing through a left ventricular outflow tract narrowed by a thick, bulging septum.

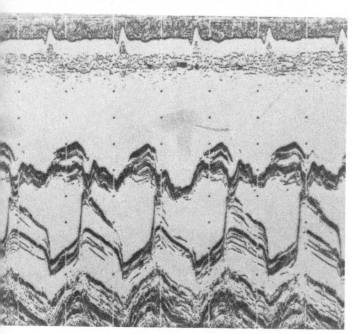

Fig. 6-18A. Mrs. Prooval's mitral valve

Celia Prooval, a 36-year-old homemaker, can no longer keep her house spotless. By midafternoon she's exhausted. Even the walk from the parking lot to the hospital has left her slightly short of breath. She recalls a childhood illness that kept her confined to bed for about four months, but no one ever told her what it was. You examine her and hear an apical, low-pitched, rumbling diastolic murmur.

THREE PATIENTS WITH DIASTOLIC MURMURS

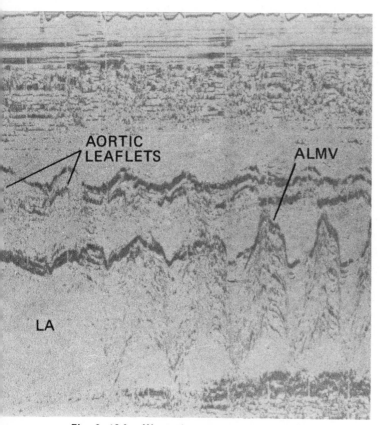

Fig. 6-19A. Wayne's aorta, mitral valve

Wayne Weede, who is 53 years old, complains of generalized weakness and a 10-pound weight loss over the last six months. This morning on awakening, he noted some weakness in his left arm and leg and came to see you in the Emergency Room. Your examination confirms a mild left hemiparesis. On auscultation, you hear a peculiar sound following the second heart sound. The resident thinks the murmur is "typical of mitral stenosis." This echocardiographic tracing was made as the sonographer directed the transducer in an arc from the aortic root (left) to the anterior mitral leaflet (right).

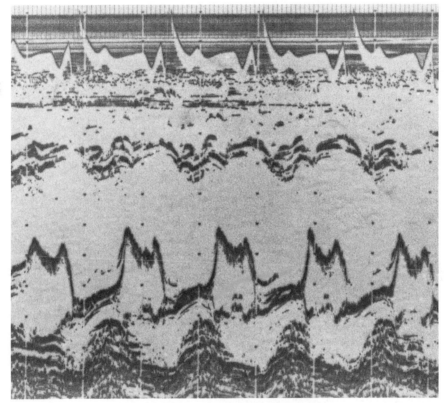

Fig. 6–20A. Dr. Shift's mitral valve

Dr. C. Redding Shift, an astronomer who is 32 years old, has come to you only at the urging of his wife. He feels well, but says he has been very aware of his heartbeat, particularly when lying down. He attributes this symptom to anxiety, related to his responsibilities at work. Your examination reveals a prominent apical impulse (but perhaps you feel it so well because of *Dr. Shift's* pectus excavatum). He also has a high-pitched blowing decrescendo diastolic murmur.

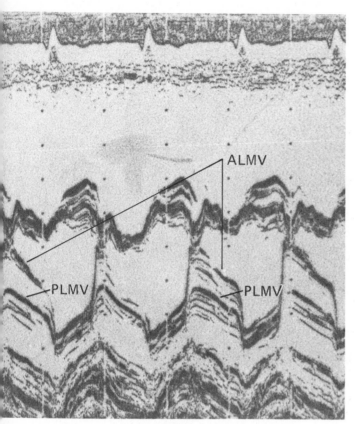

Fig. 6–18B. Mrs. Prooval—Mitral stenosis

ANSWERS

Mrs. Prooval (Fig. 6–18B) has mitral stenosis. During diastole, the thickened leaflets (ALMV, PLMV) remain open as blood slowly flows through the narrowed mitral orifice. Figure 6–18C is from another patient with the same problem. Note the markedly diminished E-F slope that is characteristic of this disease. In addition, the "A" wave, reflecting atrial contraction, is completely lost, owing to the thickened, rigid nature of the leaflet. Compare with the normal tracings (Figs. 6–10B and 6–11A), in which there is brisk opening and partial closure of the mitral leaflet during the rapid filling phase of diastole.

Note that the posterior mitral leaflet moves anteriorly during diastole in both mitral stenosis patients. This finding is seen in 90 per cent of patients with mitral stenosis and is thought to be caused by fusion of the cusps. Measurement of the height of the opening excursion and also of the closing velocity (E-F slope) of the anterior mitral leaflet may give a rough guide to the severity of the mitral stenosis.

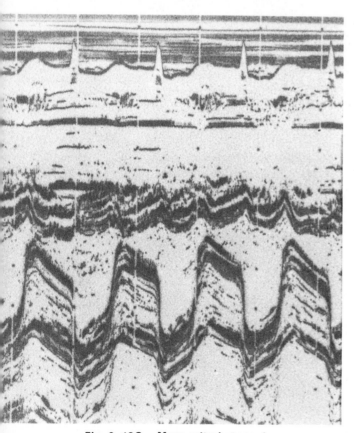

Fig. 6–18C. More mitral stenosis

ANSWERS—*Continued*

Wayne's history alerts you to suspect some cardiac problem resulting in embolic phenomena. The thoughts running through your mind as you examine him include 1) valvular vegetations, 2) left atrial thrombus, and 3) left atrial myxoma. The echogram (Fig. 6–19B) shows multiple echoes behind the mitral valve during diastole and within the left atrium during systole. This is the characteristic picture seen when a left atrial myxoma prolapses through the mitral orifice during diastole.

In Figure 6–19C, the anterior wall (AW) and posterior wall (PW) of the tumor are more clearly defined. The peculiar sound you heard following the second heart sound was, of course, the "tumor plop."

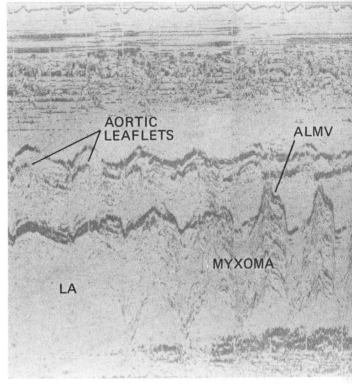

Fig. 6–19B. Prolapsing left atrial myxoma

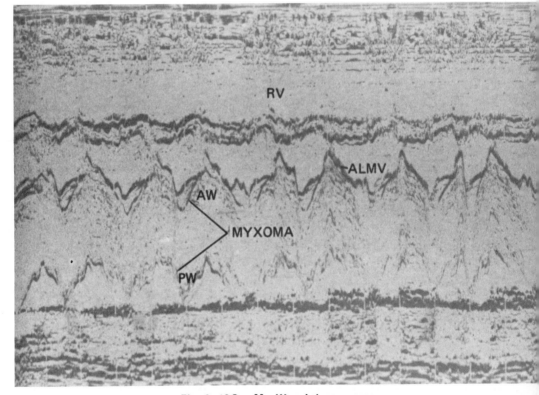

Fig. 6–19C. Mr. Weede's myxoma

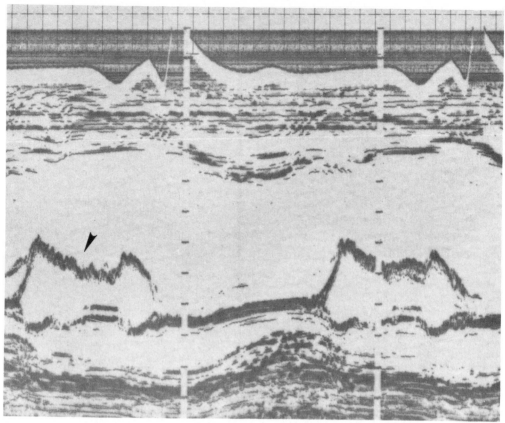

Fig. 6–20B. **High frequency oscillations, mitral valve**

ANSWERS – *Continued*

Dr. *Shift's* echocardiogram shows findings characteristic of aortic insufficiency. During diastole the regurgitant jet of blood from the incompetent aortic leaflets may strike the mitral apparatus. The anterior mitral leaflet (and sometimes the posterior mitral leaflet) then oscillates in the turbulent stream. This high frequency oscillation (arrow) is par-

ticularly well seen when the paper speed is increased so that the mitral tracing is drawn out (Fig. 6–20B). The aortic valve usually appears normal on the echocardiogram in patients with *pure* aortic insufficiency. But why should this young man have aortic insufficiency in the first place? He has no history of rheumatic fever. His serology is negative. He *could* have a bicuspid valve, but these patients usually present with findings suggestive of aortic stenosis.

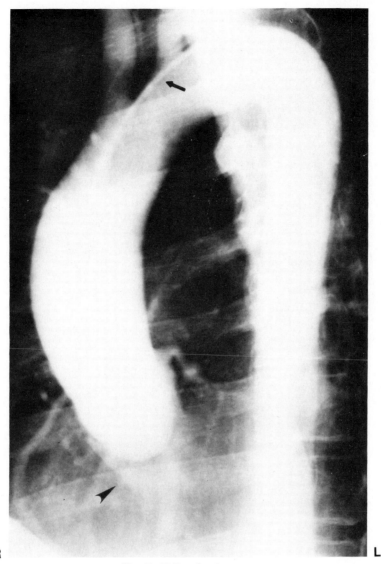

Fig. 6–20C. **Aortogram**

R   L

ANSWERS – *Continued*

The pectus excavatum gives you your clue. *Dr. Shift* has Marfan's syndrome. Patients with this disorder often have weakness of the aortic media and may present with aortic regurgitation or even with acute dissection. Myxomatous degeneration of the mitral leaflets and supporting apparatus is also common in these patients, producing significant mitral leaflet prolapse and associated mitral regurgitation. Figure 6–20C is from another patient who had an aortogram. The catheter (arrow) was inserted in the femoral artery, then its tip was moved to the aortic root. Injection of contrast material into the root shows that a small amount of the contrast (arrowhead) leaks through the incompetent aortic valve into the left ventricle. What are the linear contrast-filled vessels extending from the aortic root? The coronary arteries, of course.

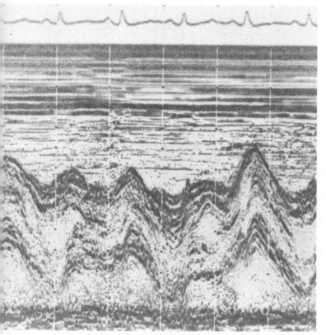

Fig. 6–21A. Frenda's left ventricle

Frenda Awl sustained a stab wound in her left chest while intervening in a quarrel between two of her clients. The 56-year-old social worker is brought to the Emergency Room in shock. You note a paradoxical pulse, start the IV's and alert the OR. A quick (and limited) echocardiographic study is obtained before the patient is moved to surgery.

TWO PATIENTS — ONE PROBLEM

While you're puzzling over the previous case, consider the echocardiogram of **Sybil Servant**, a government employee. *Sybil*, who is 38 years old, has been feeling unusually sluggish lately. While taking her history, you can't help noticing her dry skin, dull hair, and pretibial edema. Her heart sounds are faint and difficult to evaluate.

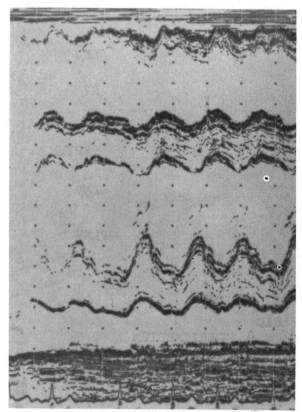

Fig. 6–22A. Sybil's left ventricle

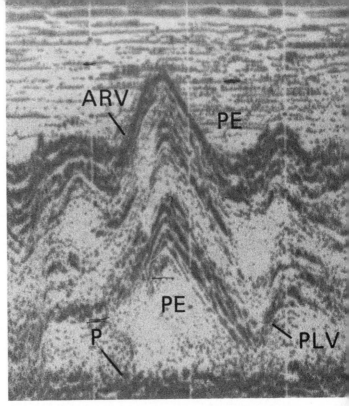

Fig. 6–21B. **Massive pericardial effusion**

ANSWERS

Both *Frenda* and *Sybil* have pericardial effusions. It's only a matter of degree. *Frenda's* effusion is so massive (over 1000 cc. of blood within the pericardial sac) that her heart gyrates ineffectively within the bag of fluid. The echocardiogram (Fig. 6–21B) shows the right (ARV) and left (PLV) ventricular walls moving together as the heart swings back and forth. The many echoes within the pericardial fluid are artefactual, owing to the high gain that was used for the study. This bizarre appearance is characteristic of massive pericardial effusion and has been described as the "Swiss Alps" appearance (Fig. 6–21C). The cardiac movement is so gross that it frequently precludes accurate echographic identification of structures other than the cardiac walls.

By the way, did you notice the electrical alternans on the ECG in Figure 6–21A? Pericardial tamponade is frequently accompanied by electrical alternans.

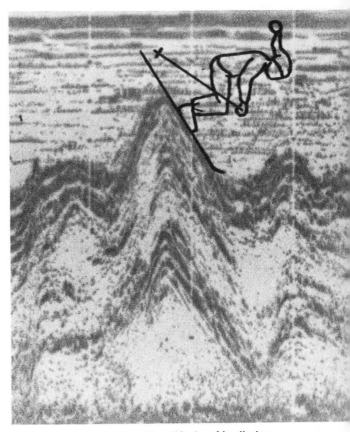

Fig. 6–21C. **"Swiss Alps" sign**

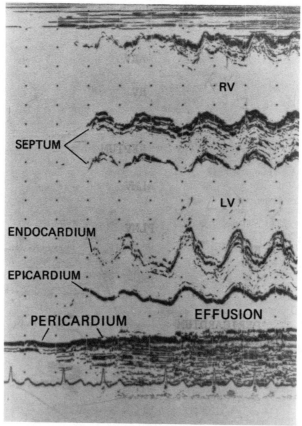

Fig. 6–22B. **Posterior pericardial effusion**

ANSWERS — *Continued*

On *Sybil's* tracing (Fig. 6–22B) the interventricular septum and posterior left ventricular wall show entirely normal motion. Behind the left ventricular wall, however, is a sonolucent area representing a pericardial effusion of about 400 cc. The pericardium is the strong echo just behind the fluid. Notice that on the left side of the picture the sensitivity setting has been dropped so low that all of the cardiac echoes disappear except the strong one from the pericardium–lung interface. This is one way to identify the exact location of the pericardium. *Sybil*, of course, had severe myxedema with secondary pericardial effusion.

NOTE: Echocardiography has been successful in identifying pericardial fluid in amounts as small as 20 cc. This technique provides only a *gross* quantitation of the actual amount of effusion, however. Serial studies on an individual patient are particularly helpful in following a change in the amount of effusion.

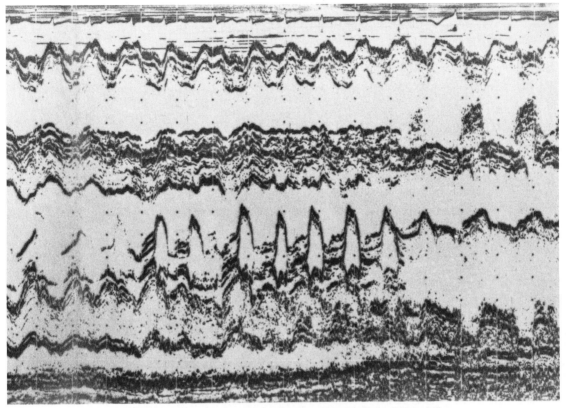

Fig. 6–22C. **Pericardial effusion. Sweep from LV to LA**

Another good way to accurately identify the location of the pericardium is to direct the transducer in an arc from the left ventricle to the aorta (Fig. 6–22C). The pericardium attaches to the left atrium at the level of the pulmonary veins, so that a pericardial effusion can only extend up to this level. Notice on the accompanying tracing how the pericardial effusion (represented by a sonolucent area behind the left ventricular posterior wall) becomes smaller and then disappears behind the left atrium. If you are wondering why the anterior mitral leaflet does not show its usual M shape, this is because the atrial contraction peak (the second peak of the M) is poorly seen in tachycardia. In atrial fibrillation, of course, it may not be seen at all. This patient also has concentric left ventricular hypertrophy. Note the thickened septum and posterior left ventricular wall (> 1.2 cm.).

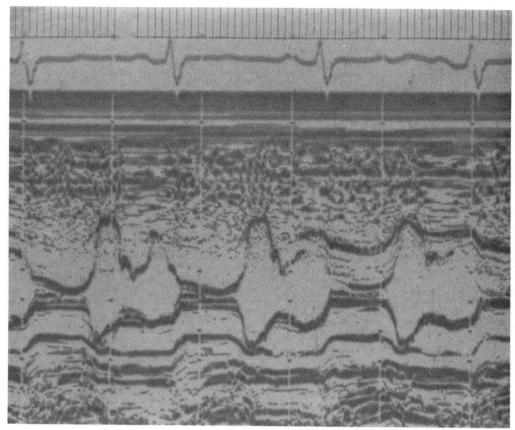

Fig. 6–23. **Normal tricuspid valve**

The Tricuspid Valve

In most normal patients, the tricuspid valve lies behind the sternum, and its motion is therefore difficult to record. In patients with right ventricular enlargement, however, it is somewhat easier to obtain a satisfactory tricuspid echogram. The motion of the normal tricuspid valve (Fig. 6–23) is similar to that of the normal mitral valve, showing a typical M-shaped configuration during diastole. Abnormalities of tricuspid valve motion have been described in patients with tricuspid stenosis and in Ebstein's anomaly. More work remains to be done, however, in detailing the configuration of the tricuspid valve motion in various disease states.

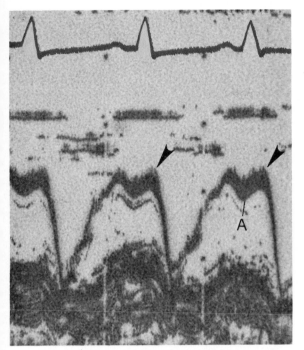

Fig. 6-24A. Normal pulmonic valve

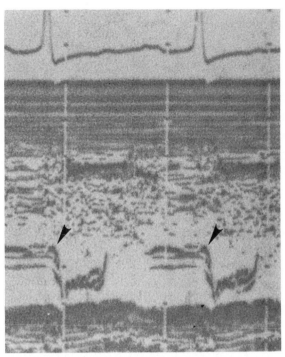

Fig. 6-24B. Pulmonary hypertension. Arrows indicate beginning of systolic opening.

The Pulmonic Valve

The pulmonic valve is also difficult to visualize in many patients. When recorded, it is usually a posterior pulmonic cusp (Fig. 6-24A) that is seen. The leaflet moves slightly posteriorly during diastole. Following atrial systole, there is a more prominent posterior displacement of the leaflet (A point), followed by systolic opening (arrows) of the valve. In patients with pulmonary hypertension (Fig. 6-24B) the diastolic slope is flat and the A point is very small or absent.

Abnormalities of pulmonic valve excursion have also been described in patients with infundibular and valvular pulmonic stenosis.

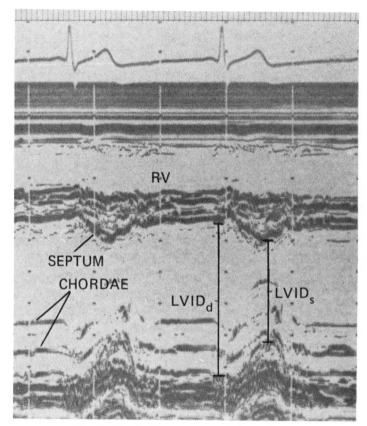

Fig. 6–25. **Left ventricular dimensions**

Left Ventricular Function

Echocardiography may also be helpful in determining the status of left ventricular function. By measuring the internal dimension of the left ventricle both in systole ($LVID_s$) and in diastole ($LVID_d$), indices of left ventricular function (stroke volume, ejection fraction, etc.) can be derived. This technique provides a noninvasive way to examine and follow up left ventricular performance. Discussion of left ventricular performance studies is beyond the scope of this text. Readers who are interested in further elucidation of these techniques are referred to the standard texts dealing with echocardiography.

Congenital Heart Disease

The use of echocardiography in the evaluation of congenital heart disease is a relatively new area of exploration. One of the greatest contributions of echocardiography is in the neonate, in whom abnormalities caused by pulmonary disease or sepsis may mimic those caused by congenital heart disease. Echocardiography can be helpful in these instances, in distinguishing cardiac from noncardiac disease.

Such congenital malformations as hypoplastic left ventricle, transposition of great vessels, Ebstein's anomaly, endocardial cushion defect, and many others also have proved themselves amenable to evaluation by echocardiography.

SUMMARY: ECHOCARDIOGRAPHY

The major uses of echocardiography today include evaluation of the following:

1. Pericardial effusion (rough quantitation)
2. Mitral stenosis (presence, degree)
3. Mitral valve prolapse
*4. Flail mitral leaflet
5. Aortic stenosis
6. Aortic insufficiency
7. IHSS
*8. Pulmonic valve (pulmonary hypertension, pulmonic stenosis)
*9. Tricuspid valve
*10. Prosthetic valves
*11. Valvular vegetations
12. Left atrial enlargement
13. Left atrial myxoma
*14. Left ventricular size and function
*15. Right ventricular enlargement
16. Atrial septal defect
*17. Congenital heart disease

---

*N.B.: Items marked with an asterisk are not discussed in detail in this chapter, but are discussed in most standard echocardiographic texts.

QUIZ AND FAREWELL TO READERS PRESENTED AS AN ACROSTIC PUZZLE

Instructions:

Acrostic puzzles are no harder than crossword puzzles and a great deal more fun.

Take our advice and Xerox the pages first so that you will have them on paper that will allow for erasures.

Then set about trying to figure out the Solving Words, and be advised that even a few of them will get you started well.

Fill in the words you figure out from their definitions (reference works help, e.g., with word V.) For example, word U, a four-letter word for the structure that regulates the size of the pupil, should be easy.

Now you can put those four letters up into the Gram in squares 129, 94, 167 and 41. When you have transferred the letters of a few more Solving Words you will find that you have enough letters to guess at the words in the Gram.

In other words ____ _Y_ must be either MY or BY, and you can fill in the other letter and transfer it *down* into the indicated Solving Word space, which may help you get *it* solved.

Working back and forth in this way is much more fun than most such puzzles because success is measured out to you in regular dollops.

No solution is printed. Those who discover the sentence in the Gram by working the puzzle will, we hope, take the message very much to heart.

They will also discover that the initial letters of the Solving Words compose an Acrostic read vertically. Hence the exclamation mark signifying the final word.

Good luck!

THE GRAM

THE SOLVING WORDS

A. $\overline{186}$ $\overline{98}$ $\overline{13}$ $\overline{131}$ $\overline{3}$ $\overline{24}$ $\overline{11}$ $\overline{15}$ $\overline{121}$ $\overline{51}$ $\overline{93}$ Mediterranean anemia.

B. $\overline{26}$ $\overline{105}$ $\overline{174}$ $\overline{187}$ $\overline{199}$ $\overline{192}$ $\overline{123}$ $\overline{200}$ $\overline{114}$ $\overline{154}$ $\overline{142}$ $\overline{61}$ $\overline{53}$ $\overline{148}$ Frequent cause of pulmonary edema in the young (2 words).

C. $\overline{180}$ $\overline{188}$ $\overline{16}$ $\overline{127}$ $\overline{12}$ $\overline{2}$ $\overline{196}$ $\overline{34}$ $\overline{90}$ $\overline{190}$ $\overline{149}$ $\overline{115}$ $\overline{191}$ $\overline{81}$ $\overline{168}$ Slipping of one part of the intestine into an adjacent part

D. A renal cyst could be so described.

| 184 | 100 | 159 | 120 | 162 | 33 | 181 | 19 | 6 | 44 |

E. What puzzles do to some people.

| 157 | 166 | 4 | 91 | 138 | 89 | 202 | 99 | 49 |

F. Their transmission and reflection have provided a new, safer diagnostic method (2 wds).

| 193 | 75 | 137 | 66 | 204 | 95 | 65 | 28 | 72 | 64 |

G. Any series of four connecting works; also a congenital heart condition.

| 118 | 163 | 79 | 133 | 77 | 130 | 42 | 216 | 134 |

H. An exclamation.

| 38 | 211 | 139 |

I. A hard, heavy and durable wood.

| 208 | 60 | 62 | 203 | 135 |

J. "There were giants in the _____ in those days" Genesis VI 4

| 201 | 144 | 150 | 194 | 109 |

K. _____ star; Polaris.

| 213 | 32 | 50 | 210 | 80 |

L. "to get the _____": comprehend implied meaning (colloq.)

| 21 | 18 | 183 | 55 | 156 |

M. An opening of relatively small size.

| 39 | 82 | 31 | 43 | 83 | 189 | 22 |

N. The basic information.

| 161 | 78 | 84 | 67 | 20 | 9 | 27 | 73 | 25 | 29 | 8 | 107 |

O. Profession of Audax Major, Vol. II

| 145 | 116 | 52 | 71 | 103 | 46 | 35 | 215 |

P. Roman ship's officer who beat time for rowers.

| 45 | 126 | 30 | 198 | 185 | 37 | 136 | 209 |

Q. Near death.

| 173 | 102 | 88 | 87 | 10 | 170 | 74 | 106 |

R. Echography.

| 143 | 158 | 206 | 54 | 14 | 165 | 1 | 152 | 69 | 125 |

S. Click beetle.

| 151 | 177 | 153 | 172 | 110 | 104 |

T. Genus of gram negative intracellular organisms transmitted to man by lice and ticks.

| 195 | 175 | 197 | 59 | 70 | 68 | 207 | 97 | 96 | 86 |

U. Regulates the size of the pupil.

| 129 | 94 | 167 | 41 |

V. Common name of the Forficulidae.

| 122 | 117 | 76 | 56 | 214 | 169 |

W. To gaze or look fixedly.

| 119 | 132 | 155 | 23 | 205 |

X. Petroleum, especially the more volatile varieties. (Word root goes back to Babylon.)

| 141 | 176 | 113 | 147 | 146 | 179 | 171 |

Y. Basic perfume used in many cosmetics (3 words).

| 17 | 212 | 92 | 160 | 124 | 40 | 57 | 47 | 101 | 48 |

Z. Hospital term for the initial history, physical exam and lab work done on a patient after admission (comp.)

| 128 | 112 | 58 | 63 | 36 | 85 | 178 | 164 | 108 | 111 | 140 |

!. Much parodied poem (1855) about the grandson of Nakomis.

| 182 | 5 | 7 |

INDEX

Note: Page numbers in *italic* type indicate illustrations.